What To Do When Your Doctor Gives Up On You

The 7 Secrets that Find the Problem,
Boost Energy, and Bring You Back to Health

Dr. Tenesha Wards, D.C., A.C.N.

DISCLAIMER

The book is for informational purposes only. Neither the publisher nor the author is engaged in rendering professional advice or services to the individual reader. The ideas, procedures and suggestions contained in this book are not intended as a substitute for consulting with your physician. All matters regarding your health require medical supervision. Neither the author nor the publisher shall be liable or responsible for any loss or damage allegedly arising from any information or suggestion in this book.

While the author has made every effort to provide accurate information at the time of publication, neither the publisher nor the author assumes any responsibility for errors or for changes that occur after publication. Further, the publisher does not have any control over and does not assume any responsibility for author or third-party websites or their content.

DEDICATION

To my mom, Lyette Lizotte Weine, who taught me never take no for an answer when you know in your heart it's a yes. Each time I gave up and failed and claimed "I can't," you'd remind me "you can and you will." Thank you for that.

And to my daughter London Wards, I pray that I instill the same fierceness in you.

To everyone suffering from illness, fatigue, and pain – JUST KEEP GOING! Your body IS designed to heal. And it will, when you give it what it needs.

Contents

ACKNOWLEDGMENTS

To the late Dr. Byron W. Schoolfield, your courage to stand up for patients with Lyme Disease in Michigan in the 1990s was courageous and heroic. I owe you my life.

Dr. Sharon Randall Himeloch, my childhood chiropractor, mentor, and friend. You taught me that a girl from Flint can grow up to be a doctor.

Healing takes a team, and boy, do I have a powerful one! Thank you to Dr. Jeannette Birnbach, Dr. Marty Ross, Dr. Deitrich Klinghardt, Dr. Wallace Taylor, Charlotte Sternkind, Patty Sprinkle, and Barbara Christman. Thanks to all of you, I was able to birth a happy, healthy baby girl, recover and still practice medicine.

Mary Schneider, Karen Hutchins, Coletta Long, and The Discovery Program Austin for your guidance on emotional healing.

To all the amazing doctors and practitioners that I've had the honor to study under the past 17 years –

Dr. John Donofrio, Dr. Joe Thomas, Dr. John Bandy, Dr. Evan Meladenoff, Dr. Stuart White, Dr. Deb Kern, Drs. Jeannette and George Birnbach, Dr. Janet Lang, Dr. Dan Khuene, Glen and Charlotte Kikel, Dr. Josh Axe, and Dr. Pete Camiolo.

Dr. Khuene and Dr. Choppa — I cherish your friendship and clinical knowledge more than you'll ever know.

To my team at Infinity Wellness Center, not only do you all run our office like a well-oiled machine, but your mission, purpose, and passion for what we do is the driving force behind our success. I am blessed to serve alongside you in the trenches.

Most of all to my husband for supporting my ever-changing, ever-growing, I-want-to-change-the-world crazy ideas. I appreciate the sacrifices you make daily so I can live my dreams. Thank you for hanging on while we take this ride called life together. But most importantly, thank you for keeping London and me well fed!

FOREWORD

As a posture-correction focused chiropractor, early in my career, I noticed that there were underlying and hidden causes that kept my patients from fully healing. Doing research, I discovered the clinical application of nutrition was the missing link. I was so thrilled about this that I started sharing my knowledge with my colleagues. As they saw similar results, I was sought out to coach and mentor hundreds of doctors across multiple disciplines on the fantastic results a well-designed nutrition program could have for their clients.

We live in a world where the miraculous yellow brick road often veers off into one dead-end promise after another. The internet allows untested theories and self-proclaimed experts to flood our minds with choices. The days of trusting a company, a license, or a professional at face value is over. Now we need to advocate for ourselves and vet our support teams for our best benefit.

And that is exciting news.

We can customize the talent of our team and trust that we are choosing from the best options and opportunities. It's easy to see public reviews, to watch other people's outcomes, and to access professionals across the globe. People, right now, are reinventing themselves and starting new chapters for their lives.

The reality of our human body is that we weren't designed to stay healthy. We were created to ADAPT to the stresses we encounter. The stresses in our lives—chemical (toxicity), emotional, and structural (injury)—are battled back by our immune response and core health. The doctors who understand this concept understand that increasing your body's health adaption response is the key to a happy, healthy, symptom-free and lovely aging lifestyle. Dr. Tenesha Wards gets it.

What I like about Dr. Wards and her book is her understanding of supporting the core principles that create the path back to health and sets up long-term success. Before identifying the seven principles that turned her own health around, she was given up on by professionals, lived through the failure of medical promises, and had to do her own sleuthing of many holistic solutions. Dr. Tenesha chose to be bold in the quest for her health and now chooses to be bold in the teaching of her discoveries.

If you feel your body is aging too quickly, your mind is reacting too slowly, or your energy is never quite enough, then step up and seize your recovery by following this unique plan.

In her book, "The 7 Secrets That Find the Problem, Boost Energy and Bring Back Your Health," she explains her process in a simple and usable plan. Get back to youthful energy and a curious mind. Make this bold choice for yourself because nobody else will. While there's no singular path, there are trustable guides and Dr. Tenesha Wards is one of them. She leads with great knowledge, courage, and a proven process that can you can implement for tremendous success in your life.

Dr. George Birnbach

Thriving in a Lyme Disease Life

"We don't always cry because we are weak, sometimes we cry because we have been strong, brave and courageous for way too long."

~Johnny Depp

My story of overcoming Lyme Disease

Overcoming debilitating health struggles with Lyme Disease as a young girl and finding the strength to not only live, but to live with passion.

My exposure to natural healing started at a young age. My mom would take me in for chiropractic adjustments as a baby for earaches and colic versus rushing to get antibiotics. She also tells a story about me at age 3, and a little bird. I found an injured baby bird and kept it in a shoebox to nurse its broken wing back to health before I let him fly off. My mom knew before I did that I'd end up in the medical field.

At age 8 or 9, my father was diagnosed with multiple sclerosis. This was traumatic for me to witness when, at one point, half his body was paralyzed and he was bedridden. I loved and cared for him at his bedside and fought with my mother when she forced me to go to school. After years of pain and suffering, he had all the mercury fillings removed from his mouth with the advice of a holistic-minded dentist. He was able to recover, function, and regain his enthusiasm for life. But nope, I only played doctor at this point and didn't quite get my calling...yet.

At age 15, I became extremely sick. I woke up one morning unable to move any joint in my body. My joints literally would not bend. I had a red, feverish rash covering most of my skin. And I hurt, everywhere. The pain was intense. I cried, a lot. Overnight I went from the natural fearlessness of a 15-year-old girl active in sports and cheerleading, to a deeply frightened teenager experiencing intense fatigue and pain. And truly thinking I may not live.

I remember my mother taking me to the doctor through the back door of the clinic. I was immediately quarantined because of the red feverish rash that covered most of my body. Doctors ran test after test with no avail. No one could figure out the source of the rash, swollen joints, and pain.

Doctor after doctor, test after test; no one knew what was wrong with me. Pumped full of drugs and steroids, I only gained weight and got worse. My fears and parents' fears escalated. One day I finally surrendered and told my mom, "Take me home, I'm going to die."

Looking back, I crossed a bridge that day. I didn't know it then, but I found the power that comes from acknowledging and naming a deep fear and letting others help you move through it. After that, my mom moved past her own fear and stepped up the research herself to find an answer. Her insistence that I be tested for Lyme disease, rare and unheard of in Michigan in the 1990s, is what saved my life. Witnessing my mother transforming her fear into action has forever made her my hero and inspiration.

I slowly started to get better. I could function to an extent and bend the joints in my hands after running them under warm water each morning. We finally found a holistic-minded doctor whose practice was similar to my practice today.

It took years of vitamins, herbs, detoxes, cleansing, genetic testing, and major gut repair to get to the healthy state I am in today – energy back, pain gone and living a life full of vitality again! As long as I follow the protocols found in this book, take care of myself and my immune system, I am able to stay in good health.

My second breakdown - my second breakdown happened after the birth of my daughter. At thirty-six years old we decided to get pregnant, knowing that Lyme can be transmitted from mother to child, I traveled all over the country working with the top Lyme Disease MDs to learn exactly what to do to ensure I did not spread this to a child. Thankfully, I ended up in Dr. Marty Ross' office in Seattle, Washington. With his guidance, I was able to conceive and carry our daughter and I am forever grateful. But it was at a price.

At this point I was living life free of any Lyme Symptoms - unless, I neglected my body. If I ate too much sugar or processed foods, stayed up too late, had increased stress, then I would feel just a bit more tired than the people around me. I have since learned this may actually be due to my poor ability to detox and genetics, but at the time I believed it was only Lyme. I was on, and had been for decades, a maintenance dose of anti-bacterial herbs and living life with tons of energy. Dr. Ross ran labs, and Lyme showed up positive. It was still in my system and I was not taking a chance. Many women at this point may choose to adopt or have a surrogate carry a child, but I chose to carry with his guidance.

We both knew the herbs I was on, the ones that kept my Lyme Disease suppressed for over 20 years, cause miscarriages and I would need to go off them. You see, in my experience with Lyme, clinically and personally, if you've had the germ in your body for longer than a year untreated - it starts to act like a virus. In the fashion of if you keep your immune system up, it stays dormant (similar to a cold sore) and you have zero symptoms. But the moment you get sick, get too stressed, eat poorly, it may rear its ugly head. Please know, this is only based on my experience and clinical research.

With my history, I took no chances and decided to move to antibiotics in order to prevent placental transmission. I felt great making the transition from herbs to antibiotics. I carried to full term, had a drug free delivery, and nursed her for a full year. I was in a state of bliss! People commented on how amazing motherhood looked on me. All was great - until I transitioned off the antibiotics when she turned one. That's when, like a house infested with termites, it all came crashing down.

I was expanding my practice with two new associate doctors, building out a new clinic, juggling a full patient load and chasing a toddler. As a chef, my husband worked many nights and weekends, and it wore on me. I could barely make it through my days. My husband and nanny took over most of the child care. I was irritable, angry, gaining weight, and fatigued to the point that some days it hurt to lift my head.

I convinced myself I was just *"mom tired."* Or, *"I will pull out of it when XYZ project was over."* I was in complete denial that I was sick. My denial almost cost me my marriage. I was difficult to be around. How could *I*, someone who helped people get well, be sick, again?? I was superwoman, juggling all the balls, spinning all the plates with grace and ease. That was how people saw me. That was how I saw myself. The shame was real. Not even my closest friends or family knew I was struggling. I covered it up at the office only to come home cranky and mean to my family, and then I would crash.

Finally, I ran tests on myself. I ran EVERYTHING! Thankfully, The Lyme had not flared up. But the prolonged antibiotics wiped out my good gut flora, despite the copious amounts of gut repair I took while on them. I was also suffering from Epstein Barr Virus, and Autoimmune Thyroiditis, Hashimoto's Disease. In other words, my immune system was gone, I had a virus that causes debilitating fatigue, and my body thought my thyroid, *my own thyroid,* was public enemy #1 and was attacking it!

Slowly, through rebuilding my immune system, gut repair, and lowering inflammation, I fully recovered. Through that experience, I created an online program to help women all over the world going through the same. The Energy Recovery System. This program is designed to help women who are not local to Austin or do not have access to this kind of care, get their lives back without the use of drugs or surgery.

My only regret (maybe) is nursing as long as I did. Forty weeks on antibiotics to carry a baby is tough enough on the body, but adding another year while I nursed was probably what caused the breakdown. However, London is healthy, shows no signs of Lyme Disease, and thriving, so it was all worth it.

If I were to advise another mother with a chronic illness, I might say nurse 3 months tops. But us mama's can be stubborn, and will sacrifice ourselves for those babies any day of the week!

Today I am happy, healthy, and once again symptom free. Is the Lyme cured? I don't know. I do know that it does not show up in my labs, I am not on any antibacterial herbs, and I feel amazing.

From my mom's example of leaving no stone unturned and the inspiration born out of my painful experiences, I now passionately work closely with clients all over the world to uncover the source of their illness, empathize with their pain and frustration, and then stay the course to help them heal.

I daily count myself blessed to be able to use my experience to help others move through their fears, pain, and fatigue, to also heal.

Dr. Tenesha Wards, D.C., A.C.N.

The Energy Recovery System

Website: www.Energy-Recovery-System.com

Instagram: https://www.instagram.com/energy_recovery_system/

Facebook: https://www.facebook.com/energyrecoverysystem/

Infinity Wellness Center

1201 West Slaughter Lane Austin, Texas 78748

Website: https://www.austinholisticdr.com

Phone: (512) 328-0505

Fax: (512) 291-7702

Email: info@austinholisticdr.com

Facebook: https://www.facebook.com/InfinityWellnessATX/

Instagram: https://www.instagram.com/infinitywellnessatx/

HEALING FROM THE INSIDE OUT

"All disease begins in the gut."

~Hippocrates

Most of us think of bacteria as harmful germs and consider them to be the major cause of sickness. We do our best to kill all germs using disinfectants and antibiotics. However, it might surprise you to know that we have trillions of beneficial bacteria present within all of us! These bacteria comprise the human microbiome, which protects our gut, health and boosts our immune system.

Healing my gut was key for me to heal both times in my life. Health truly starts in the gut. You've probably seen those yogurt commercials that say 80% of your immune system is in your gut. They are 100% right! Brilliant marketing campaign ya'll! But know, this is why it is foundational to start here.

What is the microbiome?

Microorganisms such as bacteria, fungi and viruses living in or on the human body are collectively known as the human microbiota. It consists of 10–100 trillion microbes in the gut, mainly bacteria.[1] ("Micro" means small and "biome" means a habitat of living things.)

Our microbiome has a direct effect on our health, fertility and longevity. Disturbances in our gut microbiome can lead to leaky gut syndrome, fatigue, depression, arthritis, heart disease, cancers, autoimmune diseases and even neurological disorders like dementia.

In reality, the human gut is like our second brain. It houses the enteric nervous system, which contains more than 100 million nerve cells. These cells help the GI tract digest food by regulating blood flow and intestinal secretions. However, in addition to digestion, the gut nervous system and the brain communicate with each other and affect each other's functions.[2]

For example, the gut plays a role in the management of chronic stress and disorders like depression and anxiety.[3] This is why gut-related diseases like irritable bowel syndrome can be treated with antidepressants.[4] Not recommended by the way, as that does not fix the cause... but now we see why we have so many common phrases like *butterflies in my stomach, pit in my stomach, gut feelings,* and *gut reactions.*

Leaky gut syndrome

It is an important disorder that affects not only the gut and the brain but also other organ systems. Leaky gut syndrome, rarely recognized by conventional physicians, is caused by damage to the bowel lining by toxins, poor diet, parasites, infection, alcohol, chronic stress (as we know this will eventually cause ulcers too) or medications. It leads to disruption of the tight junctions between adjacent intestinal cells and increased permeability of the gut wall. Substances such as toxins, microbes, undigested food, waste, etc. leak from the gut into the bloodstream and surrounding tissues.[5]

Increased intestinal permeability may be associated with gastrointestinal conditions such as celiac disease, Crohn's disease, inflammatory bowel disease, and irritable bowel syndrome; autoimmune diseases such as lupus, multiple sclerosis, and type 1 diabetes;[6] chronic fatigue syndrome, fibromyalgia, arthritis, allergies, asthma, acne, eczema, psoriasis, obesity, and even mental disorders like depression, anxiety, and dementia.[7] It can also interfere with the absorption of vital nutrients and minerals like Vitamin B12, iron and zinc.

Symptoms of leaky gut

Leaky gut syndrome can result in a wide variety of problems such as:

- **gastrointestinal complaints:** abdominal pain, bloating, constipation, diarrhea, gas, indigestion, heartburn.
- **neurological disturbances:** aggressive behavior, anxiety, confusion, fuzzy or foggy thinking (brain fog), mood swings, nervousness, poor memory.
- **respiratory problems:** shortness of breath and asthma and
- **other symptoms:** fatigue, poor immunity, recurrent bladder infections, recurrent vaginal infections, skin rashes, bed-wetting, chronic joint pain, chronic muscle pain, and so on.

Lab tests to confirm leaky gut

The following five tests will help you to determine if you're experiencing leaky gut syndrome:

1. **Intestinal Permeability Test (Lactulose mannitol ratio test)**

   This test is done using lactulose and mannitol, which are non-digestible sugars. After drinking a solution containing lactulose and mannitol, a urine sample is tested every 30 minutes after six hours. The presence of leaky gut is determined by their levels in the urine.[8]

2. **Food Sensitivities Test (Food Intolerance Test)**

   This test analyzes the levels of antibodies to bacteria, yeast, and commonly eaten foods in blood or saliva. Different laboratories have different names for this test depending on their specific analysis. It may also analyze all four levels of immunoglobulin G (IgG).

3. **Zonulin Test**

   Zonulin is a protein that controls the size of the openings between the gut lining and the bloodstream. High serum levels of zonulin can cause these openings to become too large and are an indicator of abnormal gut permeability. So zonulin in the stool or blood can be used as a biomarker of impaired gut barrier function.[9]

4. **Stool Tests**

   These tests can help to estimate overall intestinal health, intestinal immune function, inflammation markers, probiotic levels as well as the presence of beneficial bacteria and pathogenic bacteria, yeast, and parasites. But not any stool sample will do. It has to be a sample that detects the levels of good and bad bacteria in the gut as well as microscopic microbes. Most conventional medicine stool samples only test for parasites that you would have already seen in the toilet – tapeworms, pinworms, etc. We prefer the GI Map stool test – it shows good and bad levels, microscopic parasites, fungus, and viruses in the GI tract.

5. **Organic Acids Test**

   The organic acids test provides a detailed analysis of your health by providing information about vitamin, mineral and amino acid deficiencies, levels of antioxidants and bacteria, oxidative stress damage, detoxification, yeast and bacterial overgrowth, and many other markers.[10]

Leaky gut healing tips

There is no standard solution to treat leaky gut. Instead, you may require dietary and lifestyle changes to suit your personal situation. However, there are four basic steps to heal leaky gut **The Four R's to a Healthy Gut:**[11]

1. **Remove the Bad:** Eliminate foods that damage the gut including inflammatory foods such as processed foods, added sugar, GMOs, refined oils, alcohol, caffeine, synthetic food additives and conventional dairy products. Minimize exposure to environmental toxins in tap water, pesticides, cleaning material, cosmetics, and so on. You may also need to review your use of medications such as NSAIDs and antibiotics. Consult your physician about medications that may be causing gut

damage. Remove any parasites, unwanted bacteria, fungus and viruses.

2. **Replace with the Good:** Eat gut-healing foods anti-inflammatory foods including:

   - fermented vegetables such as sauerkraut and kimchi
   - sprouted seeds like chia seeds, flaxseeds and hemp seeds.
   - steamed vegetables
   - **fruits (low glycemic /** in moderation)
   - cultured dairy like yogurt and kefir
   - bone broth
   - **healthy fats** like egg yolks, **avocados,** ghee and coconut oil
   - **foods** containing **omega-3 fatty acids** like grass-fed beef, lamb, and wild-caught fish like salmon

3. **Repair the Damage:** Soothe and nourish your gut's lining, seal any leaks, reduce inflammation and encourage the production of healing fatty acids. Take digestive enzymes to improve digestion and specific leaky gut supplements and herbs like butyric acid, **L-glutamine,**[12] licorice root, marshmallow root,[13] aloe vera juice, and shilajit.[14]

4. **Reinoculate:** Restore the balance of the microbiome with prebiotics and probiotics. **Prebiotics** are high-fiber foods such as whole grains, greens, vegetables, fruits, beans, and lentils that act as food for human microflora and boost "good" bacteria in the gut. **Probiotics** present in foods such as yogurt and sauerkraut are live microorganisms that maintain and improve the normal microflora (good" bacteria) in the body. In addition, probiotics and prebiotics are also available as dietary supplements.

Next steps:

If you suspect you have leaky gut syndrome, you need to seek medical help right away. Unfortunately, leaky gut does not heal on its own; it gets progressively worse. You need to find out if you have leaky gut – get the GI Map test run.

If you do, treat it ASAP by removing inflammatory foods and adding the healing foods and one or more of the above Repair herbs.

GETTING RID OF THE HANGRY, HOW FOOD CREATES MOOD

"You better cut the pizza in four pieces because I'm not hungry enough to eat six."

~Yogi Berra

We've all been there – Hangry! Hangry is a blend of hungry and angry and it means to be irritable or angry because of hunger. According to Dr. Michael Knight, assistant professor of medicine at George Washington University School of Medicine and Health Sciences, "Hunger is a signal that the brain needs more fuel.

It's triggered when the level of nutrients in our bloodstream begins to drop. One of the most common emotions is anger – and that's why, many times, when we become hungry, we become irritable."[15]

If you are frequently hangry two to three hours after a meal, it might be because of hypoglycemia (low blood sugar). Hypoglycemia is sometimes a common symptom of **prediabetes**, which may develop into type 2 diabetes.[16] But it also stresses out the endocrine system to have your blood sugar dip too low, leading to adrenal gland stress.

The pancreas and its relation to the endocrine system

The pancreas is an abdominal organ that secretes digestive enzymes into the small intestine and hormones directly into the bloodstream. Its digestive enzymes are trypsin, chymotrypsin, amylase, and lipase. Amylase digests carbohydrates, lipase digests fats, and trypsin and chymotrypsin digests proteins.

The three hormones secreted by the pancreas are insulin, glucagon, and somatostatin.

- **Insulin** lowers the level of glucose in the blood by moving glucose into muscles and other tissues.

- **Glucagon** raises the level of glucose in the blood by stimulating the liver to release its stores.
- **Somatostatin** prevents the other two hormones from being released.[17]

Usually, insulin and glucagon work together to keep blood glucose levels balanced. However, in diabetes, the pancreas either doesn't produce enough insulin or the body doesn't respond properly to insulin (insulin resistance). This causes an imbalance between the effects of insulin and glucagon.

In type 1 diabetes, the pancreas isn't able to produce enough insulin and so blood glucose becomes too high unless insulin is injected.

In type 2 diabetes, the body does not respond effectively to insulin, leading to high blood glucose levels.[18]

Type 1 diabetes typically occurs before the age of 20.

Type 2 diabetes is the more common form of diabetes. It is usually seen in people over 40, especially if they're overweight and sedentary.

Prediabetes is a condition in which your blood glucose levels are higher than normal. However, they are not high enough to be diagnosed as diabetes. Prediabetes usually occurs either when the pancreas isn't making enough insulin to keep blood glucose in the normal range or due to insulin resistance. If they don't correct its underlying causes, people with prediabetes will ultimately develop type 2 diabetes.

Prediabetes is diagnosed if the fasting blood glucose level is between 100 mg/dL and 125 mg/dL or the blood glucose level is between 140 mg/dL and 199 mg/dL two hours after a glucose tolerance test.[19]

The National Diabetes Statistics Report of the Centers for Disease Control and Prevention (CDC) reports the following sobering facts about diabetes and prediabetes.

- **Diabetes:** 30.3 million people have diabetes (9.4% of the US population). Out of them, 23.1 million people have been diagnosed and 7.2 million people are undiagnosed.
- **Prediabetes:** 84.1 million adults aged 18 years or older have prediabetes (33.9% of the adult US population).[20]

This means that one in ten of us have diabetes and one in three have prediabetes!

The Role of Stress in Diabetes

During times of stress, the body ensures that there is enough glucose in the blood for the fight or flight response. It does this by secreting less insulin and more glucagon and adrenaline so that more glucose is released from the liver into the blood. It also secretes more growth hormone and cortisol, which reduces the sensitivity of body tissues to insulin. As a result, more glucose is available in the blood. Therefore, blood sugar is more difficult to control during times of stress such as infections, other illnesses or prolonged or intense emotional stress.[21] As you can see, stress can cause blood sugar dysregulation and blood sugar dysregulation can cause the body to stress!

Signs and Symptoms of high blood sugar versus low blood sugar

High blood sugar (hyperglycemia)

The symptoms of high blood glucose levels are variable and depend on its duration and intensity as well as the organs affected. They include:

- increased thirst
- increased urination
- increased hunger
- blurred vision
- drowsiness
- nausea
- tingling numbness and weakness of lower limbs
- reduced balance and coordination

- delayed wound healing, especially in the feet and legs
- decreased endurance during exercise[22]

Unfortunately, many people with diabetes may have no symptoms at all and their diabetes may only be detected during a random blood test or due to symptoms caused by diabetic complications.

Low blood sugar (hypoglycemia)

The symptoms of hypoglycemia can often be much more troublesome and dangerous, and may even be life-threatening. Therefore, one of the principles of prevention and treatment of diabetes is to minimize the frequency and intensity of hypoglycemia and to correct it as soon as possible.

Mild hypoglycemia may cause the release of adrenaline (indicating the adrenals glands are stressed) into the blood leading to:

- nervousness
- sweating
- hunger
- shaking
- faintness
- heart palpitations

Severe hypoglycemia may result in confusion, weakness, fatigue, dizziness, headaches, slurred speech, blurred vision, seizures, and coma. These symptoms are because of a reduced supply of glucose to the brain. Severe and prolonged hypoglycemia may permanently damage the brain.[23] That's why low blood sugar is much more dangerous than high blood sugar.

Labs to confirm blood sugar dysregulation

Doctors check blood glucose levels in people who have symptoms of diabetes such as increased thirst, urination or hunger. Additionally, doctors may check blood glucose levels in people who have disorders that can be complications of diabetes, such as frequent infections, foot ulcers, and yeast infections.

Blood glucose

A blood sample is taken after you have fasted overnight to measure your fasting blood glucose level. Fasting blood glucose levels should not be higher than 100 mg/dL. A second blood sample may be taken two hours after you have eaten to measure your postprandial blood glucose level, which should be less than 140 mg/dL. (However, each lab has its own range of normal values that may vary slightly.)

Hemoglobin A1c (HbA1c)

Hemoglobin A1c is also called glycosylated or glycolated hemoglobin. Hemoglobin is the red, oxygen-carrying protein molecule in red blood cells. When blood is exposed to high blood glucose levels for a while, glucose attaches to the hemoglobin and forms glycosylated hemoglobin. The hemoglobin A1c level (the percentage of hemoglobin that is glycosylated) reflects average blood glucose levels in the past 2 to 3 months. This is because red blood cells in the human body survive for 8-12 weeks before renewal.

Below is the range of Hemoglobin A1c we like to follow in functional medicine. The Normal Range and Prediabetic Range are a little lower when we look at it from a prevention perspective.

HbA1c Percentage

Normal	Below 5.8%
Prediabetes	5.8% to 6.4%
Diabetes	6.5% or over

If your hemoglobin A1c level is 6.5% or more, you have diabetes. (This is the same in both functional and conventional medicine.)

Two large-scale studies – the UK Prospective Diabetes Study (UKPDS) and the Diabetes Control and Complications Trial (DCCT) – demonstrated that improving HbA1c by 1% reduced the risk of diabetes-related complications in the eyes, nerves and kidneys by 25%.[24]

Oral glucose tolerance test

This test is not routinely used to detect diabetes. It is usually done for screening pregnant women for gestational diabetes. In this test, a blood sample is taken after overnight fasting to determine the fasting blood glucose level. More blood samples are then taken over the next 2 to 3 hours after drinking a solution containing a large, standard amount of glucose to determine whether the glucose in the blood rises to abnormally high levels.[25]

Natural ways to regulate blood sugar

If untreated, people with diabetes mellitus may experience many serious, long-term complications, including nerve damage, kidney disease, blindness, lower limb amputations, stroke, and even death.[26]

If you have type 1 diabetes, you need to take insulin injections. If you have type 2 diabetes, your traditional doctor will most likely advise you to take antidiabetic medications and insulin.[27] However, it is possible to prevent or even reverse type 2 diabetes with diet and lifestyle changes such as a healthy diet, regular exercise, and weight loss.[28]

Four Steps to Regulate Blood Sugar

1. **Eat unprocessed or minimally processed foods**

   The first step in the prevention and reversal of diabetes is to eat healthy and nutritious food such as vegetables, lentils, beans, millets, fruits, berries, nuts, seeds, wild-caught fish, organic chicken, and grass-fed beef. These foods are anti-inflammatory, high in fiber and have a low glycemic index, which means they are converted into sugar much more slowly after being eaten. Following a structured healthy diet also helps to lose weight and reverse diabetes permanently.

2. **Eliminate or minimize foods that raise blood sugar levels and cause inflammation**

   If you want to reverse diabetes, you have to avoid or minimize processed foods containing refined sugar, processed grains, hydrogenated oils, alcohol, and dairy products. And needless to say, you have to stop smoking.

3. **Take supplements and herbs**

   The following supplements are especially useful in diabetes.

   - **Alpha Lipoic Acid** improves insulin sensitivity and especially useful in diabetic neuropathy[29]
   - **Cinnamon** reduces plasma glucose, LDL cholesterol and triglyceride levels[30]
   - **Bitter Melon Extract** reduces insulin resistance and complications of diabetes[31]
   - **Chromium** improves sensitivity to insulin[32]
   - **Fish oil** contains omega-3 fatty acids, which improve insulin action and reduces inflammation[33]
   - **Coenzyme Q10** is useful in diabetes because of its antioxidant action and may reduce fasting plasma glucose and hemoglobin A1C levels[34]
   - **Ginseng and Gymnema** are herbs that suppress appetite and boost metabolism. Also, it helps to reduce weight and blood sugar[35]

4. **Regular exercise**

Daily exercise helps to prevent or reverse type 2 diabetes, overall health, and quality of life.[36] If you are physically unfit and haven't exercised recently, consult your doctor before starting any exercise regimen.

Next steps:

When is the last time you got checked for high blood sugar? If it's been more than a year, you need to get it done right away. As already mentioned, 7.2 million Americans with diabetes are undiagnosed.

Diabetes is a silent killer because it may not display any symptoms for months or even years. In this case, knowledge is power and forewarned is forearmed because the sooner you detect it, the sooner you can reverse it.

Walking the pH Tightrope – Alkalize to Live

"He that takes medicine and neglects diet wastes the skill of the physician."

~Chinese Proverb

Your body's pH balance is the level of acids and alkalis in your blood. pH means the "potential of hydrogen" or the measure of the hydrogen ion concentration of a solution.[37]

The pH scale ranges from 1 to 14.

- seven is neutral
- pH less than 7 is acidic
- pH greater than 7 is alkaline or basic

The difference between adjacent numbers on the pH scale represents a tenfold difference in acidity. For instance, a pH of 5 is 10 times more acidic than a pH of 6 and 100 times more acidic than a pH of 7.

Body pH—acid versus alkaline

An important property of our blood is its degree of acidity or alkalinity. Blood is normally slightly basic, with a normal pH range of 7.35 to 7.45. Usually, the pH of our blood is maintained at around 7.4.[38]

The pH of our stomach is around 1.5 to 3.5. The pH of saliva and urine is also slightly acidic, usually between 6.4 to 6.8 in a healthy individual.

When the acid level in your blood is too high, leading to a blood pH lower than 7.35, it's called acidosis. When the alkali level in your blood is too high, leading to a blood pH higher than 7.45, it's called alkalosis

Conditions like chronic stress, poor diet, lack of mineral-rich foods, smoking, drug use (both prescription and recreational) and illness can cause gradual depletion of mineral reserves and lead to acidosis. Many diseases and disorders are associated with an acidic condition – diabetes, obesity, allergies, constipation, morning sickness, acid reflux, osteoporosis, gout, migraines, cataracts, stroke, cancer, and so on.

Signs and symptoms of low pH

Symptoms of low pH in the body include chronic fatigue, muscle and joint pain, sleep problems, air hunger, itchy skin and irritable bowel.

There are three types of acidosis:

1. **Respiratory acidosis** is caused when your lungs are not able to remove enough carbon dioxide when you exhale. Conditions that could lead to respiratory acidosis include disorders like asthma, emphysema, pneumonia, neurological disorders that affect breathing and sleep medications.

   If you have respiratory acidosis, you may feel extremely drowsy, tired, confused and have a headache. If left untreated, it can lead to coma or death.

2. **Metabolic acidosis** is excess acid in the body that originates in the kidneys. It occurs when your body can't get rid of excess acid or loses too much alkali. It is caused by

   • severe vomiting or diarrhea leading to low sodium bicarbonate in your blood
   • diabetic ketoacidosis leading to excess ketones in your blood

- alcohol misuse, cancer, and seizures leading to excess lactic acid
- renal tubular acidosis caused by the inability of the kidneys to excrete acid in the urine and
- ingesting toxic substances, such as methanol, antifreeze and aspirin (in large doses)

Symptoms of metabolic acidosis include severe fatigue, nausea and vomiting.

As with respiratory acidosis, metabolic acidosis, if left untreated, can result in coma or death.

3. **Dietary acidosis** has been recognized as a legitimate form of acidosis only recently. This is important in the functional nutrition world for the prevention of disease. It is caused by eating a highly acidic diet that puts undue stress on the body and increases the risk of chronic disease.[39]

Lab tests for pH

The pH of the urine is an accurate reflection of the pH of the entire body. The body's acid/alkaline balance can be measured by testing the urine using pH paper. I have all my new patients perform this test for 7 consecutive days after their first visit with me and report back the average.

First-morning urine pH test

First-morning urine is defined as the first urination after 5 AM. It is tested to determine whether the pH is acid or alkaline. If the urine pH is acidic (pH below 6.8), it indicates that the body is in a state of distress due to insufficient minerals.

Evening urine pH test

After the pH of the first-morning urine is consistently in the alkaline range for at least 2 weeks, the next step is to test the evening urine pH. It should be measured just before dinner. If both urine tests are within the recommended range, it means you are sufficient minerals in the body.

Depending on your symptoms, your doctor may ask for additional tests such as:

- arterial blood gas for oxygen and carbon dioxide levels and blood pH
- basic metabolic panel to check kidney function
- glucose and ketone levels, if you have diabetes

Natural ways to alkalinize your body

Acidic foods may increase the risk of inflammation, which is linked to chronic diseases such as cancer[40] and heart disease.[41] It is believed that bacteria, viruses, fungi, and cancers have a hard time growing in a basic environment.[42] Acidic foods may also be linked to acid reflux, kidney stones, low bone density, and chronic pain.

Your body usually maintains pH balance within a narrow range. However, if your doctor finds that your pH balance to be abnormal through blood and urine testing, they will do additional tests to determine the exact cause. Once the cause is discovered, you'll be given a treatment plan to correct it and get your body's pH balance back to normal.

If your urine is too acidic (below 6.4), you may be advised to take an alkaline diet consisting of:

- fresh vegetables, including potatoes
- most fruits
- beans and lentils
- whole grains, such as millet, quinoa, and amaranth
- fats like olive oil, avocados, nuts, and seeds
- herbs and spices, excluding salt, mustard, and nutmeg

- herbal teas
- soy, such as soybeans, miso, tofu, and tempeh
- unsweetened yogurt and milk
- add a mineral supplement to your regimen

You will also have to limit or avoid foods that tend to cause acidity in the body such as:

- grains
- sugar
- processed foods
- sodas and other sweetened beverages
- certain dairy products
- red meat
- high-protein foods and supplements
- high-phosphorus drinks such as beer

An alkaline diet has the following health benefits:

- Fruits and vegetables improve the potassium/sodium ratio, which may improve bone health, reduce muscle wasting, and mitigate hypertension and strokes.
- An alkaline diet increases growth hormone leading to improvement in cardiovascular health, memory, and cognition.

- It also increases intracellular magnesium, which is required for proper functioning of many enzyme systems.[43]

Next steps:

An alkaline diet is extremely helpful in hard-to-treat conditions like leaky gut syndrome, Lyme Disease, chronic conditions like diabetes, and hormonal disorders like adrenal fatigue.

In addition to highly alkaline foods in your diet – try this tonic in the morning: one teaspoon of baking soda and one teaspoon of lemon juice in water first thing in the morning. Also, adding minerals at night will increase morning urine pH to help alkalize your body.

Maximize Hormones for All Day Energy

"To control your hormones is to control your life" ~Barry Sears

Overview of the endocrine system

The endocrine system is like a symphony, it consists of a group of glands and organs that secrete various hormones that all have to work together in harmony. Hormones are chemical substances that control and coordinate activities in the body.

- **Exocrine** hormones such as bile and pancreatic digestive enzymes are released through ducts

- **Endocrine** hormones such as cortisol, thyroxine, and adrenaline are released directly into the bloodstream

The Human Endocrine System[44]

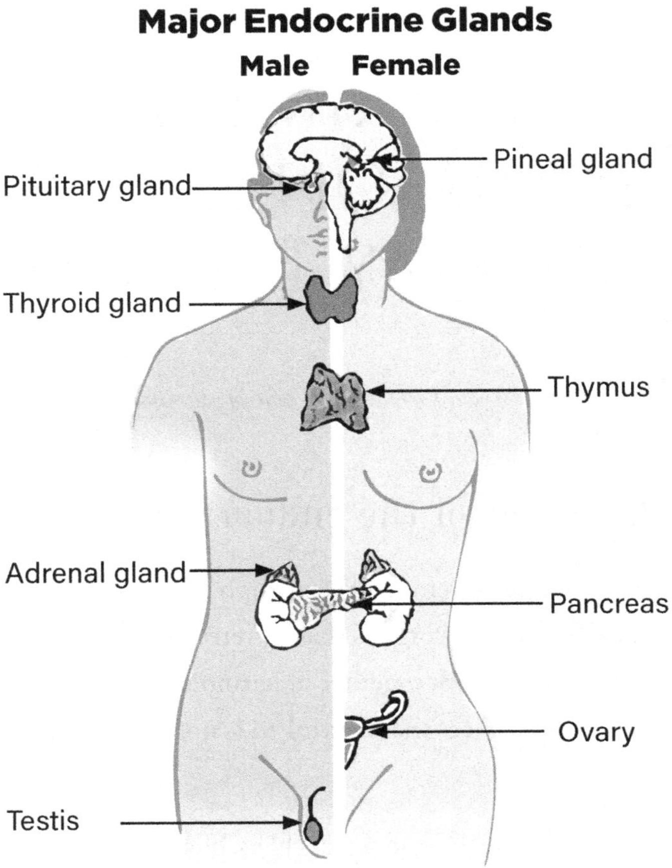

Major Endocrine Glands
Male   Female

Pituitary gland

Pineal gland

Thyroid gland

Thymus

Adrenal gland

Pancreas

Ovary

Testis

The major glands of the endocrine system are:

- hypothalamus
- pituitary gland
- thyroid gland
- parathyroid glands
- islet cells of the pancreas
- adrenal glands
- testes in men and ovaries in women
- placenta in women (during pregnancy)

The pancreas secretes endocrine hormones like insulin and glucagon as well as exocrine digestive enzymes like trypsin, amylase, and lipase.[45]

Endocrine Controls

Many endocrine glands are controlled by the interplay between the hypothalamus and the pituitary gland, which is called the hypothalamic-pituitary axis. The hypothalamus secretes several hormones that control the pituitary gland. In turn, the pituitary gland controls the functions of other endocrine glands. Therefore, it is sometimes called the master gland, or in Yoga the third eye. Spiritually many consider that gland the connection to your higher self or creator. It knows and controls all. The blood levels of other endocrine hormones will signal the pituitary to decrease or increase the secretion of its hormones (feedback loop).

For example, if blood levels of thyroid hormone are low, the pituitary gland releases thyroid stimulating hormone (TSH), which signals the thyroid gland to secrete more hormones. If blood levels of thyroid hormone get too high, the pituitary decreases the amount of TSH, which then signals the thyroid to decrease secretion of thyroid hormone.

Other factors can also control endocrine function. For example, rising blood sugar levels stimulate the pancreas to produce more insulin.[46]

Major Endocrine Hormones and Their Functions

Hypothalamus

- **Corticotropin-releasing hormone:** Stimulates the release of adrenocorticotropic hormone
- **Gonadotropin-releasing hormone:** Stimulates the release of luteinizing hormone and follicle-stimulating hormone
- **Growth hormone-releasing hormone:** Stimulates the release of growth hormone
- **Somatostatin:** Inhibits the release of growth hormone, thyroid-stimulating hormone, and insulin

- **Thyrotropin-releasing hormone:** Stimulates the release of thyroid-stimulating hormone and prolactin

Pituitary Gland

- **Corticotropin (adrenocorticotropic hormone - ACTH):** Controls the production and secretion of hormones by the adrenal glands
- **Growth hormone:** Controls growth and development and promotes protein production
- **Luteinizing hormone and follicle-stimulating hormone:** Control reproductive functions, including the production of sperm and semen in men and egg maturation and menstrual cycles in women. They also control male and female sexual characteristics (including hair distribution, muscle formation, skin texture and thickness, voice, and perhaps even personality traits)
- **Oxytocin:** Causes muscles of the uterus to contract during childbirth and after delivery and stimulates contractions of milk ducts in the breast, which move milk to the nipple
- **Prolactin:** Starts and maintains milk production in the ductal glands of the breast (mammary glands)

- **Thyroid-stimulating hormone:** Stimulates the production and secretion of hormones by the thyroid gland
- **Vasopressin (antidiuretic hormone):** Causes kidneys to retain water and, along with aldosterone, helps control blood pressure

Thyroid Gland

- **Thyroid hormones: T3 and T4** Regulate the rate at which the body functions (metabolic rate)
- **Calcitonin:** Tends to decrease blood calcium levels and helps regulate calcium balance

Parathyroid Glands

- **Parathyroid hormone:** Controls bone formation and the excretion of calcium and phosphorus

Adrenal Glands

- **Cortisol:** Has widespread effects throughout the body, especially anti-inflammatory action. Maintains blood sugar level, blood pressure, and muscle strength. Helps control salt and water balance
- **Aldosterone:** Helps regulate salt and water balance by causing the kidneys to retain salt and water and excrete potassium

- **Epinephrine and norepinephrine:** Stimulate the heart, lungs, blood vessels, and nervous system
- **Dehydroepiandrosterone (DHEA):** Has effects on bone, mood, and the immune system

Pancreas

- **Insulin:** Lowers the blood sugar level and influences the metabolism of sugar, protein, and fat throughout the body
- **Glucagon:** Raises the blood sugar level

Digestive Tract

- **Cholecystokinin:** Controls gallbladder contractions that cause bile to enter the intestine. Stimulates release of digestive enzymes from the pancreas
- **Ghrelin:** Controls growth hormone release from the pituitary gland. Causes sensation of hunger
- **Glucagon-like peptide:** Increases insulin release from the pancreas

Kidneys

- **Erythropoietin:** Stimulates red blood cell production
- **Renin:** Controls blood pressure

Ovaries

- **Estrogen:** Controls the development of female sex characteristics and the reproductive system
- **Progesterone:** Prepares the lining of the uterus for implantation of a fertilized egg and readies the mammary glands to secrete milk

Testes

- **Testosterone:** Controls the development of male sex characteristics and the reproductive system

Placenta

- **Chorionic gonadotropin:** Stimulates ovaries to continue to release progesterone during early pregnancy
- **Estrogen and progesterone:** Keep uterus receptive to fetus and placenta during pregnancy

Adipose (Fat) Tissue

- **Leptin:** Controls appetite
- **Resistin:** Blocks the effects of insulin on muscle[47]

Endocrine Disorders

Endocrine hormones serve as messengers that regulate and control various functions throughout the body. Endocrine disorders involve either

- hyperfunction, that is, too much hormone secretion
- hypofunction, that is, too little hormone secretion

Disorders may result from a problem in the gland itself or because of too little or too much stimulation by the hypothalamic-pituitary axis. Sometimes the body's immune system attacks an endocrine gland and decreases hormone production (autoimmune disorders such as Hashimoto's thyroiditis). Finally, tumors originating in the endocrine glands can either produce excess hormones or destroy normal glandular tissue.

Examples of endocrine disorders include

- Hyperthyroidism
- Hypothyroidism
- Diabetes
- Addison disease
- Adrenal fatigue
- Cushing disease

- Acromegaly
- Disorders of puberty and reproductive function

Doctors usually measure levels of hormones in the blood to tell how an endocrine gland is functioning. Sometimes blood levels alone do not give enough information about endocrine gland function, so doctors may measure hormone levels:

- at certain times of the day or more than once a day (such as cortisol) in saliva
- after giving a stimulus or suppressor (such as a sugar-containing drink, a drug or a hormone that can trigger or block hormone release)
- after having the person take an action (such as fasting)

Endocrine disorders are often treated by replacing a hormone that is deficient or reducing levels of a hormone that is excessive. However, sometimes the cause of the disorder can be treated. For example, a tumor involving an endocrine gland may have to be removed.[48]

Effects of Aging on the Endocrine System

Levels of most endocrine hormones decrease with aging. However, some hormones do not decrease and some may even increase. Irrespective of hormone levels, endocrine function may decline with age because hormone receptors become less sensitive.

Endocrine hormones that decrease with aging:

- estrogen (leads to menopause in women)
- testosterone (usually decrease gradually in men)
- growth hormone (may lead to decreased muscle mass and strength)
- melatonin (may lead to loss of normal sleep-wake cycles)

Endocrine hormones that remain unchanged or decrease slightly:

- cortisol
- insulin
- thyroid hormones

Hormones that may increase include epinephrine, in the elderly, norepinephrine, parathyroid hormone, follicle-stimulating hormone, and luteinizing hormone.

Though hormone replacement therapy might be beneficial in older people with decreased function, it does not always reverse aging or prolong life. And estrogen replacement in some older women may be potentially harmful.[49]

Signs and symptoms of endocrine imbalance

Some of the most common signs and symptoms of hormone imbalances include:

- fatigue
- **insomnia**
- depression and anxiety
- digestive problems
- appetite changes
- unexplained weight loss or weight gain
- **low libido**
- infertility and **irregular periods**
- hair thinning and **hair loss**

Symptoms of hormonal imbalance and the type of disorder or illness they cause depend on the glands that are affected. For example, symptoms of diabetes caused by insulin resistance may include fatigue, changes in appetite, nerve damage and problems with eyesight.

Some specific problems associated with some of the most common hormonal imbalances include:

- **Adrenal fatigue:** fatigue, brain fog, muscle pains, anxiety, depression, insomnia, and reproductive problems

- **Diabetes:** weight gain, nerve damage (neuropathy), higher risk for vision loss, fatigue, dry mouth, and skin problems
- **Hypothyroidism:** fatigue, anxiety, irritability, weight gain, digestive problems, constipation, and irregular periods
- **Hyperthyroidism:** weight loss, anxiety, thinning hair, trouble sleeping, heart palpitations, diarrhea, and malabsorption
- **Polycystic Ovarian Syndrome (PCOS):** weight gain, infertility, acne, abnormal hair growth, and risk of developing diabetes
- **Low testosterone:** fatigue, erectile dysfunction, infertility, weight gain, muscle loss or weakness, and mood-related problems[50]

Testing for endocrine imbalance

Testing for endocrine disorders is not simple because the endocrine system is complex and interconnected. Therefore, problems with any one of the different kinds of glands in the endocrine system may result in changes to another, making it more difficult to pinpoint the exact problem.

A comprehensive assessment is essential because different endocrine disorders will result in different symptoms. Urine tests, blood tests, salivary tests as well as imaging technology and other tools may be used to:

- measure the levels of various hormones in the patient's body
- test normal function of one or more endocrine glands
- identify a tumor or other abnormality in the endocrine glands
- confirm the diagnosis based on history, physical examination and other means[51]

Symptoms of endocrine disorders may be nonspecific and insidious. Therefore, biochemical diagnosis is essential by measuring the blood levels of the peripheral endocrine hormone, the pituitary hormone or both.

As most hormones have circadian rhythms, these tests need to be made at different times of the day. For example, a cortisol blood test may be done once in the morning when cortisol levels are at their highest, and then around 4 pm. A cortisol saliva test is usually done late at night when cortisol levels are lower.[52]

Adrenal stress index—saliva test

The Adrenal Stress Index (ASI) is one of my favorite tests for looking at possible adrenal fatigue. It measures adrenal function by measuring cortisol and five other hormones in five saliva samples over 24 hours.

- **Cortisol**: Evaluates stress response
- **Insulin**: Investigates blood sugar control and insulin resistance
- **DHEA/DHEA-S**: Determines how other hormones may be affected by stress
- **Total secretory IgA (sIgA)**: Evaluates the toll of stress on immunity
- **17-OH Progesterone**: Determines underlying causes of abnormal cortisol levels
- **Wheat gluten sIgA**: Identifies immune response to gluten

The Adrenal Stress Index can be useful to identify and assess adrenal fatigue, sleep disorders, metabolic syndrome, allergies, autoimmune disorders, Cushing's syndrome, Addison's disease, etc.[53]

Saliva hormones

Saliva testing is used for measuring hormones like cortisol, estrogen and testosterone. The collection process is convenient, noninvasive and painless. You can collect saliva at home at specific times, which is important for accurately measuring hormone levels.

Steroid hormones in the blood are almost fully bound to carrier proteins (95-99%). They are inactive and unavailable to target tissues in this form. Saliva testing is more directly related to specific symptoms of excess or deficiency of the hormone because it measures the amount of bioavailable unbound hormone in the saliva. Ample scientific evidence proves that saliva testing is as accurate as conventional blood testing. Therefore, saliva testing is the preferred option for hormone testing and monitoring hormone therapy.[54]

Thyroid and pituitary lab tests

Lab tests for thyroid

Thyroid-stimulating hormone (TSH) and thyroid hormones (T3 and T4) levels in the blood are tested. A low level of thyroxine and a high level of TSH may indicate hypothyroidism. High levels of thyroxine and low or zero levels of TSH may indicate hyperthyroidism. You may also have to undergo thyroid antibody tests to diagnose Hashimoto's thyroiditis, an autoimmune disease that causes hypothyroidism or Graves' disease, an autoimmune disease that causes hyperthyroidism.[55]

Often a traditional practitioner will not dig deep enough to order the thyroid antibodies, so be sure to ask for them! These are antithyroglobulin antibodies and thyroid peroxidase antibodies. This could be a huge miss in figuring out your case. Addressing the autoimmunity/Hashimoto's thyroiditis entails lowering inflammation to stop your body from attacking its own thyroid. This is a very different process than just balancing thyroid hormones.

Lab tests for pituitary glands

These tests help to detect excess or deficient hormones and to diagnose specific disorders and their severity. They can also be used to monitor the effectiveness of treatment. Testing usually includes the hormones that the pituitary produces as well as the hormones of the endocrine glands that the pituitary stimulates such as

- Prolactin
- LH and FSH
- TSH and thyroid hormones
- ACTH and cortisol
- GH and IGF-1

Pituitary hormones levels in the blood may:

- be relatively constant (e.g. TSH)
- change over the course of a day (e.g. cortisol)

- change over a cycle (e.g. FSH and LH during the menstrual cycle)
- increase in specific situations such as ACTH as a response to stress or prolactin in women who are breastfeeding

Because of these variations, suppression or stimulation tests may be used to measure pituitary hormonal changes after a person takes medications to suppress or stimulate the production of these hormones. For example, a water deprivation test may be used to diagnose diabetes insipidus.[56]

How to balance the endocrine system

Hormonal imbalances are caused by a combination of factors such as your diet, medical history, genetics, stress levels and exposure to toxins from your environment. Some of the major contributors to hormonal imbalances include:

1. high levels of inflammation caused by a poor diet and a sedentary lifestyle
2. overweight or obese
3. autoimmunity
4. genetic susceptibility
5. chronic stress, and insufficient sleep and rest

6. toxicity (exposure to pesticides, toxins, viruses, cigarettes, excessive alcohol, and harmful chemicals)[57]

7. food allergies and leaky gut: New research proves that gut health plays a significant role in hormone regulation. If you have leaky gut syndrome or a lack of beneficial probiotic bacteria lining in your intestinal wall, you're more susceptible to hormonal problems, including diabetes and obesity. That's because inflammation usually starts in the gut and then affects all other systems[58]

Conventional treatment for hormonal disorders usually includes

- replacing a deficient hormone by replacement of the peripheral endocrine hormone or
- suppressing excessive production of a hormone with radiation therapy, surgery, and drugs that suppress hormone production[59]

Unfortunately, conventional treatment has a high risk of side effects. Also, they provide symptomatic relief but do not address the root cause, and lead to lifelong dependence on prescription hormones and drugs. However, you can use these natural ways to balance your hormones:

Healthy fats such as avocados, coconut oil, and wild-caught salmon. They are essential for hormone production and also lower inflammation, boost metabolism, and promote weight loss.

Adaptogenic herbs such as ginseng, astragalus, eleuthero root (Siberian ginseng), ashwagandha, holy basil and rhodiola are useful in adrenal fatigue and other endocrine disorders. They tend to increase your energy when you are tired and produce a calming effect when you feel anxious and stressed.[60] Basically, adaptogenic herbs allow you to ADAPT to life!

Essential Oils may have a role to play in some hormone disorders. For example, fennel oil relaxes your body, improves your digestion and reduces inflammation; lavender oil helps to deal with anxiety, depression and insomnia; clary sage may relieve PMS and PCOS symptoms and thyme oil helps to treat PCOS, menopause, depression, insomnia and hair loss.

Supplements can help to address nutritional deficiencies that contribute to hormonal imbalance. For example, probiotics can help to repair leaky gut, and evening primrose oil helps to relieve premenstrual and PCOS symptoms.[61]

Protomorphogens

They are nutrients derived from the cell substance of glands and direct cell repair and maintenance. They have regenerative capabilities and provide a template for the body to create better and healthier cells.

Protomorphogens revitalize sick tissues such as the thyroid, adrenal, heart, kidney, pancreas, nerves, liver, bones, digestive organs, reproductive organs, and the immune system. They are tissue-specific because each organ has its specific cellular instructions on how to produce and heal within its own cellular substance.

Every cell in our body has immune capabilities. Our immune system has two primary functions: immunity and regulation of cellular growth and repair. Dr. Royal Lee and others began researching cell growth in the 1930s. Dr. Lee explained the complex relationships between normal and abnormal cell growth, immune response, and autoimmunity. He formulated supplements of animal-derived products that could normalize and heal the immune system and every organ type.

Dr. Lee called these supplements protomorphogens (PMGs), meaning primary form or structure. A PMG is the specific cellular material extracted from the cell nucleus containing the nucleoprotein. The nucleoprotein contains genetic DNA and RNA, which regulates the structural regeneration of the cell.

In an unhealthy body, there may be mineral deficiency, improper coding, insufficient protein availability and poor intercellular function. By adding dietary PMGs and complementary nutrients, our ability to create and support healthy tissue becomes greatly enhanced. So, PMGs can reprogram the formation of our organs and direct their growth and healing.[62]

Avoid endocrine disruptors

They are chemicals that interfere with our body's endocrine system and produce a range of adverse effects. Endocrine disruptors are found in many products of daily use, including food, toys, cosmetics, detergents, pesticides, plastic bottles, metal food cans, and flame retardants. Research shows that endocrine disruptors may pose the greatest risk during prenatal and early postnatal development when organ and neural systems are forming.

Endocrine disruptors can:

- mimic naturally occurring hormones in the body like estrogens, androgens, and thyroid hormones and cause overstimulation

- bind to receptors and block the endogenous hormone from binding, which causes failure of normal response. Examples of chemicals that block hormones are anti-estrogens and anti-androgens
- interfere with the production or elimination of natural hormones, for example, by altering their metabolism in the liver[63]

Avoid the use of these top 14 endocrine disruptors:

1. BPA (plastics)
2. Dioxin (insecticide)
3. Atrazine (insecticide)
4. Phthalates (new electronics)
5. Perchlorate (chlorines)
6. Fire Retardants
7. Lead
8. Arsenic
9. Mercury
10. PFCs (perfluorinated chemicals)
11. Organophosphate pesticides
12. Glycol ethers
13. Sulfates
14. Phthalates

Next steps:

Hormonal disorders are difficult to diagnose and treat without specialized help. If you think you have a hormonal disorder like adrenal fatigue or a thyroid problem, have your hormones tested, and balanced. Start supporting the endocrine system with adaptogenic herbs if you are under stress.

YOUR DAILY DETOX, FORTIFY YOUR DEFENSES

If our goal is to destroy the world—to produce global warming and toxicity and endocrine disruption—we're doing great.

~William McDonough

It is said that there is only one disease that afflicts us—though it has a thousand names. In actuality, all illnesses originate from too many toxins in the body.

Our foods, drugs, personal products and everyday items contain more than a staggering 100,000 chemicals, with about 1000 new chemicals introduced every year.[64] Avoiding toxins is just not possible. The good news—

detoxification does not have to be a tremendous amount of difficulty or drama. Simple daily detox actions can fit in your life with very little effort to gain extraordinary increases in your natural defenses.

The latest Centers for Disease Control and Prevention (CDC) National Report on Human Exposure to Environmental Chemicals (2015) tested for 265 different industrial chemicals and found increasingly worrisome levels in our blood and urine.[65,66]

Toxins and free radicals

Toxins are poisonous substances that are produced by the metabolic activities of a living organism. They are usually very unstable, harmful and may induce antibody formation. We have been using natural toxins for killing weeds, insects, and animals since ancient times. For example, South American tribes tipped their arrows with curare, which they extracted from a vine.[67]

Free radicals are reactive atoms or groups of atoms that have one or more unpaired electrons. They are produced in the body by natural biological processes or introduced from an outside source (such as tobacco smoke, toxins or pollutants).[68]

Our bodies produce free radicals naturally during breathing, digestion, and other natural functions.[69] These free radicals are not harmful; in fact, they are necessary for the proper functioning of our immune system. They are used by the liver for detoxification and by the white blood cells to defend against infections.

Normally, free radicals are balanced by antioxidants in the body. However, this balance can be disturbed by excess production of free radicals and/or low intake of antioxidants.

The main sources of free radicals include:

- Environmental/air pollutants
- unfiltered water
- tobacco, alcohol, and drugs
- medications including antibiotics
- unhealthy diet
- radiation
- excessive exercise
- prolonged stress

Free radicals are dangerous because they are unstable molecules. Electrons exist in pairs but free radicals have an unpaired electron. So, they rob other cells and compounds of one of their electrons. In turn, these cells or compounds rob electrons from other cells and compounds. This leads to a chain reaction in the body and the rise of more and more free radicals, which damage DNA, cellular membranes, enzymes, and blood.

The damage done by free radicals in the body is known as oxidation. Oxidation is the same process that rusts metal and the amount of oxidation in the body is a measure of oxidative stress.

Oxidative stress can affect every organ in the body and lead to conditions such as diabetes, arteriosclerosis, heart disease, cancer, asthma, accelerated aging, Alzheimer's disease, and leaky gut syndrome.

Detox organs

Detoxification is our body's process of getting rid of toxic substances. This natural detox process is going on continuously – 24/7, 365 days of the year. This is done by our body's six detox organs: the liver, lungs, kidneys, colon, skin, and lymph.

- **Liver:** It cleans and filters every ounce of blood and breaks down harmful chemicals so that they can be eliminated easily including alcohol, drugs, and chemicals in food, air, personal care products, and our environment.

- **Lungs:** Your lungs get rid of carbon dioxide, allergens, fumes, mold, and airborne toxins.
- **Kidneys:** The two kidneys filter waste and toxins from the blood into the urine including by-products of protein metabolism as well as excess sugar, salt, and fluid.
- **Colon (large intestine):** It excretes the solid waste that is left after all the nutrients have been absorbed. It contains the microbiome, protective bacteria that break down food and play an important role in immunity.
- **Skin:** The skin gets rid of waste through sweat and oil glands.
- **Lymph:** The lymphatic system is composed of lymph flowing through lymphatic vessels and lymph nodes. It parallels the blood circulation and removes bacteria, viruses, and other toxins from the circulation.

Each organ eliminates waste products and metabolites that are by-products of our natural metabolic process. These organs are also called the detoxification pathways through which toxins are detoxified and removed from the body.

Genetics and detox

"Genes load the gun but lifestyle pulls the trigger."

~*Bart Penders*

Many genes play a role in the complex process of detoxification. We produce, repair, and switch off DNA through a process called methylation.[70]

Methylation is one of the main detoxification pathways that takes place in every cell, tissue and organ, billions of times per second. The most important gene influencing this methylation process is called the MTHFR gene. It provides instructions for the production of an enzyme called MTHFR (methylenetetrahydrofolate reductase), which helps to process two nutrients—folate and methionine. MTHFR converts folate into its active form (methylfolate) and homocysteine into methionine.

Both folate and methionine support the body in making and repairing DNA. Variations in the MTHFR gene affect the activity of the MTHFR enzymes. Low methylation affects the production of a molecule called glutathione, which is the most important antioxidant in your body. MTHFR variations affect each person differently. Either there are no symptoms at all or there may be serious long-term health problems.

A mutation in the MTHFR C677T and/or MTHFR A1298C genes has been found in 30 to 50 percent of people, which is inherited and transmitted from parent to child.[71]Around 14 to 20 percent of the population may have a more severe MTHFR mutation. However, research is still pending on the medical conditions that are affected by MTHFR gene mutations, including fatigue, digestion, brain function, cholesterol levels, and endocrine functions.[72]

The only way to know the status of your MTHFR gene is genetic testing. The MTHFR gene and other genes that influence detoxification work at different rates due to genetic defects. Genetic testing will help you to understand the variations in your genes, your detox deficiencies, and the corrective actions you need to take to allow your genetic pathways to express properly (with the guidance of your doctor).

Lab tests for liver function— AST, ALT, GGT

The liver helps the body to digest food, store energy, and detoxify poisons. Liver function tests are blood tests that determine how well the liver is working. They are done if you have symptoms of liver disease or as part of a regular checkup.

Liver function tests include testing for:

- Bilirubin
- Albumin and total protein (TP)
- Prothrombin time
- Enzymes that are found in the liver, including aspartate transaminase (AST), alanine transaminase (ALT), alkaline phosphatase (ALP), and gamma-glutamyl transpeptidase (GGT)[73]

Aspartate transaminase (AST)

When the liver is damaged, it releases the AST enzyme into the bloodstream. An AST blood test measures the amount of AST in the blood and helps to detect liver damage or disease. It is also called SGOT test.[74]

Alanine transaminase (ALT)

High levels of ALT in the blood can indicate a liver problem even before you have signs of liver disease such as jaundice. An ALT blood test is helpful in early detection of liver disease. It is also called SGPT test.[75]

Glutamyl transpeptidase (GGT)

Both alkaline phosphatase (ALP) and GGT are elevated in liver disease. In functional medicine, we also consider gallstones. But only ALP will be elevated in bone disease. Therefore, if the GGT level is normal in a person with a high ALP, the cause of the elevated ALP is likely to be bone disease.[76]

How to detox the body

Antioxidants counteract free radicals by donating an electron to free radicals. Glutathione is considered the most important "master" antioxidant and is the liver's major weapon. It's created from the amino acids cysteine, glycine and glutamic acid. Other major antioxidants include vitamins A, C and E, D, beta-carotene, bioflavonoids, CoQ10, selenium, zinc, copper, and manganese.

Our ability to produce antioxidants in the body declines with age. Antioxidants protect us from age-related diseases caused by free radicals and inflammation. In addition, regular exercise, good sleep, adequate water, and wholesome relationships help us to live longer, healthier, and more energetic lives.

The American Heart Association, Cleveland Clinic and the Mayo Clinic recommend getting antioxidants naturally from unprocessed whole foods instead of supplements. Such foods also contain protein, vitamins, minerals, and fiber—all of which work together synergistically. Therefore, the benefits of these foods are greater than the sum of their parts. In addition, we must minimize the use of unnecessary medications and pollutants, and reduce excessive physical and emotional stress.[77]

Detox/Cleanse

We live in a toxic world and are constantly exposed to toxins, heavy metals, pesticides, synthetic hormones, plastics, chemicals and electromagnetic frequencies in food, air, water, medicines, and dental work. In addition, we may experience tremendous mental and emotional stress at home and at work.

Detox diet

Usually, our natural detoxification system can eliminate most toxins from the body. However, we can boost this natural detox process with a detox diet. A good detox diet provides all of the important nutrients while excluding all the unhealthy food, chemicals, and toxins for a limited period. It consists of:

- Whole and unprocessed or minimally processed foods, including fruits, vegetables, beans, nuts, seeds, and sprouts
- natural detox foods such as berries, beets, grapefruit, brussels sprouts, and chia seeds

- healing herbs and spices like turmeric, cinnamon, basil, cumin, paprika and parsley
- drinking half your weight in ounces

During the detox period, exclude all sugar, artificial sweeteners, and unhealthy processed food from your diet. Ensure that you get at least eight hours of sleep at night so that your body can be refreshed and rejuvenated. Do some gentle exercise daily but make sure you don't overdo it. Finally, minimize your stress with meditation, journaling, and relaxing with your family and friends. Most important, consult your doctor before starting your detox diet.[78]

Chinese medicine recommends a detox diet during every change of season. For optimum health, you should detox once every quarter for a period of 21 days (that is, three weeks in every three months).

Next steps:

Chronic fatigue is often caused or worsened by toxicity from stealth infections, molds, harmful chemicals, heavy metals, allergies, and/or stress. If you are a poor detoxer, you need to consider genetic testing. (We recommend the detox panel by GX Sciences).

Knowing your genetic detoxification status and liver function is helpful to know when to help your body detox.

For a simple way to initiate your body's detoxification and to purge toxins, start the day with a teacup of warm water, adding a wedge of lemon or lime juice and a pinch of cayenne. Adding this liver tonic every morning will boost your liver function, digestion, and metabolism.

Purchase a water filter to filter out toxins in your drinking water.

EXTERMINATE INFECTIONS

"The germ is nothing, the terrain is everything."

~Antoine Béchamp

An overview of microbes

This chapter hits home having dealt with many pathogens. I was an opportunistic host for these germs two different times in my life. By changing my terrain, I healed. It reminds me of the saying - it's not the rosebush that's the problem if it won't bud, it's the soil.

Microbes are tiny organisms that include bacteria, viruses, fungi, algae, and parasites. They far outnumber humans and they will be here long after we are gone!

They play a major role in virtually all disease processes—ranging from infectious diseases such as cholera, malaria, and TB to chronic conditions like Lyme Disease and Epstein Barr Virus. Infectious diseases are still a leading cause of death in developing countries.

Microbes can be divided into two groups:

Normal flora, the friendly bacteria that inhabit your gut and skin, have developed a symbiotic relationship with you; they get what they need without causing harm. In many cases, they actually help us by inhibiting the growth of other potential pathogens or by breaking down substances in the gut to provide essential nutrients.

Pathogens are disease-causing microbes. An infection is when pathogenic microbes invade and multiply in the body. Disease is when the infection causes damage to the individual's system and affects its functioning. However, an infection does not always result in disease.[79]

Stealth pathogens

They are microbes that can survive undetected for years in the human body. The most common stealth pathogens are:

- **Epstein–Barr virus (EBV)** is a virus responsible for infectious mononucleosis.

- **Babesia** is a malaria-like parasite spread by ticks that can infect red blood cells to cause babesiosis.

- **Bartonella** are gram-negative bacteria responsible for cat scratch disease and trench fever. Bartonella can be spread by ticks, fleas, biting flies, and lice.

- **Borrelia burgdorferi** causes Lyme disease, typically through the bite of a tick.

- **Mycoplasma** are the smallest free-living organisms. Their unique feature is that they don't have cell walls, which makes them resistant to many conventional antibiotics and treatments. Mycoplasma are a common cause of walking pneumonia and are commonly found among those with autoimmune diseases such as rheumatoid arthritis and multiple sclerosis.[80]

These stealth pathogens can sit dormant in your body, then something else may stress your immune system and they see the opportunity to rear their ugly head! Next thing you know, they are causing symptoms like fatigue, brain fog, joint pains, and poor sleep, and may persist if your immunity is low. All these symptoms are caused by pro-inflammatory cytokines such as interleukin-6, tumor necrosis factor-alpha, and Interleukin-1 beta. Over time, this low-grade inflammation can lead to joint damage, leaky gut, fibromyalgia, leaky blood-brain barrier, atherosclerosis, obesity, insulin resistance, and Alzheimer's disease.

Diagnosis and treatment are based on the patient's history of their symptoms, clinical examination, and laboratory findings. Lab tests include IgG and IgM levels (antibodies) to these stealth pathogens. The best protection from these chronic infections is a strong immune system supported by antimicrobial herbs and a healthy lifestyle.[81]

Bacteria, viruses, fungi, parasites and algae

Bacteria are microscopic organisms that live in soil, the ocean and atmosphere and also within our bodies. Some bacteria are useful, such as those that turn milk into yogurt or help with our digestion (microbiome). However, they can also be destructive by causing diseases like pneumonia and gastroenteritis. And antibiotic resistance has become one of the biggest public health challenges of our time.[82]

Viruses are microscopic infectious agents that replicate only inside the living cells of an organism. Viruses can infect all types of life forms, from animals and plants to microorganisms, including bacteria.[83] Common diseases caused by viruses include common cold, chickenpox, and influenza as well as serious diseases such as AIDS, Ebola virus disease and EBV.

Fungi include microorganisms such as yeasts and molds as well as mushrooms. Since the 1940s, fungi have been used for the production of antibiotics such as penicillin. Some fungi can cause diseases in humans such as aspergillosis and candidiasis, which may be fatal if untreated. Other fungi can cause local infections such as ringworm and athlete's foot. People with low immunity are particularly susceptible to infection by fungi.[84]

Parasites are tiny organisms that live on or in a host organism and gets its food from or at the expense of its host.

NOTE: YOU DO NOT HAVE TO HAVE RECENTLY VISITED A THIRD-WORLD COUNTRY TO GET AN INTESTINAL PARASITE.

I literally see them every week in patients who picked them up at salad bars, biting their nails, letting their dogs lick their mouth and eating sushi—just to name a few sources.

There are three main classes of parasites that can cause disease in humans:

- **protozoa** such as entamoeba, giardia, balantidium and plasmodium
- **helminths** such as tapeworms and roundworms
- **ectoparasites** such as ticks, fleas, lice, and mites that attach or burrow into the skin and remain there for relatively long periods (weeks to months)[85]

Lyme disease

Lyme disease is caused by the bacterium Borrelia burgdorferi and is transmitted to humans through the bite of infected blacklegged ticks. **It is the most common tickborne infectious disease in the U.S.**[86] And, in my opinion, it's the most underestimated and least talked about rising disease of our time. It is truly becoming an epidemic. Up to 300,000 Americans are diagnosed with Lyme disease every year, according to the U.S. Centers for Disease Control and Prevention (CDC). Lyme is often under-diagnosed and under-reported, so many experts believe the number of infected is actually much higher.

Lyme disease symptoms may start with flu-like symptoms, fatigue, muscle pain, headaches, and joint pain. Over time, the symptoms may worsen and turn into a chronic inflammatory response that is similar to an autoimmune illness.[87] Lyme disease can be difficult to diagnose since many of its symptoms closely mimic other health problems and autoimmune disorders. *That is why Lyme is called "The Great Imitator".*

Contrary to popular belief, there are cases of Lyme disease in almost every state every year, with many more cases going undiagnosed because symptoms are non-specific and testing is difficult and unreliable.

Untreated Lyme disease can lead to serious infections, joint degeneration, arthritis, heart and blood vessel complications, nerve damage and endocrine dysfunction and neurological disorders.[88]

According to the CDC, "Patients treated with appropriate antibiotics in the early stages of Lyme disease usually recover rapidly and completely. Antibiotics are commonly used for oral treatment include doxycycline, amoxicillin or cefuroxime axetil. This often works IF the infection is treated quickly – within 3-6 months of infection. Patients with certain neurological or cardiac forms of illness may require intravenous treatment with drugs such as ceftriaxone or penicillin."

Although antibiotics can help many people to overcome Lyme disease, they may not resolve symptoms fully and may be associated with side effects and complications such as digestive problems, loss of appetite, brain fog, poor memory, chronic fatigue, pain, body numbness, seizures, and even death in rare cases.[89]

Therefore, it is vital to strengthen the immune system and oftentimes continue treatment with anti-microbial herbs when dealing with Lyme disease to reduce a chance of it turning into a chronic infection.

Prevention of Lyme disease is the first and foremost step. Use a natural insect repellent and perform daily tick checks to prevent getting Lyme disease. Wear light-colored clothing when outside and tuck your pants into your socks to prevent skin contact. After you have been in tick habitat, get out of your clothes quickly, thoroughly check your entire body and remove attached ticks immediately. Once attached, ticks do not wash off in the shower and must be removed properly with tweezers. Finally, put your clothes into the washer/dryer immediately. (The dryer kills ticks by drying them out.)[90]

As mentioned above, maintaining a strong immune system is critical for overcoming Lyme disease. Many symptoms of Lyme are caused by an immune response in the body, which means the state of your immune system determines how intense symptoms will be.

You can prevent and treat Lyme disease by improving your overall immunity.

- Take care of allergies and other illnesses that might be contributing to your symptoms because it's possible that Lyme disease is not the only thing affecting your health.

- Track your symptoms and note the things that cause symptom flare-ups such as a lack of sleep, infections, stressful events and a poor diet.

- Make sure your diet is healthy and nutritious and avoid foods that will cause inflammation.

- Take suitable supplements such as vitamin D, omega-3 fish oils, and adaptogenic herbs.

- Get plenty of rest and balance activity with rest.

- Get some exercise daily, even if it is short stroll and low-intensity activities like stretching, yoga and tai chi.

- Reduce emotional stress. Practice stress-relieving techniques regularly like deep breathing, meditation, journaling, reading and exercising. Equally important is to reach out to family and friends for support and social activities.

- If you have an active infection, look into antimicrobial herbs such as Otoba Bark extract (Otoba parvifolia), Cat's Claw (Uncaria tomentosa), Grapefruit Seed Extract or a product called Biocidin LSF (helps with neurologic Lyme) or Biocidin (best for joint pain and fatigue). I like Biocidin as it also breaks down biofilms, which are protective barriers that germs build to protect themselves. I also like to pulse these herbs when a patient meets max dose such as 5 days on, 2 days off. Always consult a Lyme literate practitioner to know which herbs are best for your body and situation, I don't suggest walking this journey alone.

- If a person gets worse due to a Herxheimer die-off reaction, we'd need to readdress their detoxification pathways and oftentimes slow down on the anti-microbial herb dose.

Epstein-Barr virus infection (EBV)

The Epstein Barr virus (EBV) is also called human herpesvirus 4. It is one of eight herpes viruses that infect humans. The Epstein Barr virus spreads through intimate contact through bodily fluids, especially saliva. After infection, all herpesviruses remain latent within host cells and may reactivate at any time.[91]

The Epstein Barr virus mainly causes mononucleosis (mono) but it has also been linked to seven autoimmune diseases: celiac disease, type 1 diabetes, multiple sclerosis, juvenile idiopathic arthritis, rheumatoid arthritis, systemic lupus erythematosus, inflammatory bowel disease, including Crohn's disease and ulcerative colitis.

EBV has also been linked to the development of cancers such as Hodgkin disease, B lymphoproliferative disease, Burkitt's lymphoma, nasopharyngeal carcinoma, and nose and throat cancers.

Many people become infected with EBV in childhood. EBV infections in children usually cause no symptoms or the symptoms are mild. EBV infection symptoms in teenagers or adults get better in two to four weeks. However, some people may feel fatigued for several weeks or even months. After an EBV infection, the virus becomes latent (inactive) in the body and it may reactivate in future. People with weakened immune systems are more likely to develop chronic active Epstein Barr virus and symptoms such as chronic fatigue, swollen lymph nodes in the neck, enlarged spleen and liver.[92]

Diagnosing EBV infection is difficult because the symptoms are non-specific and similar to other illnesses. EBV infection can be confirmed with a blood test that detects antibodies to EBV-associated antigens. About nine out of ten adults have antibodies that show that they have a current or past EBV infection.[93]

You can help protect yourself by not kissing or sharing drinks, food or personal items, like toothbrushes, with people who have EBV infection.

With EBV being a virus, the goal is to become stronger than the virus, so it will become dormant in your system and you no longer have fatigue and other symptoms. The best treatment for EBV is supportive and immune-boosting measures such as:

- drinking fluids to stay hydrated
- getting plenty of sleep and rest
- eat small and frequent meals
- eat nutrient-dense foods such as leafy green and other vegetables, green smoothies, fruits, berries, avocado, olive oil, coconut oil, nuts, and seeds.
- take anti-viral herbs such as monolaurin and Pau D'arco, and other supplements that can support your immune system such as vitamin C, vitamin D, echinacea, licorice root, and probiotics

Candida (Yeast)

Candidiasis is a fungal infection caused by yeasts that belong to the genus Candida. The most common infection is caused by Candida albicans. Candida normally lives on the skin and inside the body. It can be found in the mouth, throat, gut, and vagina without causing any problems. However, candida can cause infections if they grow out of control or enter deep into the body into the bloodstream or organs like the kidney, heart or brain. Candida auris is an emerging fungus that presents a serious global health threat because it causes severe illness in hospitalized patients and is resistant to multiple antifungal drugs.[94] Oftentimes traditional practitioners do not take Candida too seriously until it reaches this point. I like to address it much sooner.

Earlier symptoms of candidiasis include chronic fatigue, mood swings, oral thrush, sinus infections, intestinal distress, brain fog, hormonal imbalance, skin and nail fungal infections, and recurrent vaginal and urinary tract infections.[95]

Treatment of candida infection depends on the severity and site of infection.

The following supplements may be useful:

1. Pau D'arco and antifungal herbs
2. Vitamin C boosts the immune system
3. Lavender oil, clove oil, oregano oil and myrrh oil (topically or internally) are all useful in the treatment; of candida infection. However, they should be taken internally for not more than 30 days[96]

Genetic testing

A genetic mutation in MTHFR (methylenetetrahydrofolate reductase) may lead to high levels of homocysteine in the blood and low levels of folate and other vitamins. MTHFR can play a part in how your body can detox germs as well as the NOS2 gene. This gene regulates the generation of nitric oxide (NO) by nitric oxide synthase (iNOS). This pathway is involved in complex immunity, anticancer and anti-infective mechanisms. Alteration in the level and activity of the NOS2 gene may be responsible for the susceptibility, severity and outcome of genetic as well as infectious diseases.[97]

People with a genetic variation (SNP or single nucleotide polymorphism) in this gene are more prone to infections. The big question is: Why are people getting bit by the same ticks and one person is infected with the disease and another isn't? Could it be because of this gene defect? I believe so.

Everyone with stealth pathogens should consider genetic testing. If positive, we may add anti-infective herbs or extra immune-boosting nutrients to their regimen as a preventive measure.

Next steps:

Chronic infections are notoriously hard to pinpoint and even harder to eradicate. Thanks to my personal experience with Lyme disease and EBV and with hundreds of my patients, we are confident that we can help you overcome these infections once and for all.

KEEPING IT
ALL TOGETHER

"Eat food. Not too much. Mostly plants."

~Michael Pollan

This is where you have to be conscious of what goes in your body, what activities are too much for you, and what your thoughts are. To keep it all together, to ensure your fatigue, pain, or illness does not return, is work. I've had patients ask me when will they will ever be done working on themselves? My answer – not this life time!

Healthy Foods

A healthy diet consists of low-glycemic carbohydrates in the form of fruits and vegetables, healthy fats, and clean protein sources.

The three simple steps for a healthy diet are:

1. **Get rid of refined sugars and grains from your diet**

   Excessive consumption of sugar has been linked to leaky gut, chronic fatigue, obesity, insulin resistance, diabetes, ADHD, heart disease, and cancers. However, not all carbs are unhealthy. Low-glycemic carbohydrates in the forms of fruits and vegetables have high amounts of fiber, enzymes, vitamins, minerals, and antioxidants that detoxify your cells and boost energy and health.

2. **Replace unhealthy fats with healthy fats**

   Unhealthy fats such as trans fats from partially hydrogenated oil and saturated fats can contribute to chronic fatigue, obesity, diabetes, heart disease, stroke, and cancer. Good fats including unrefined vegetable oils (such as olive, avocado, flax and coconut oils), nuts, seeds, and fish are essential for production of hormones and development of the brain. They may also help to fight inflammation and boost cellular healing.

3. **Replace unhealthy proteins with healthy proteins**

Hundreds of studies link the consumption of commercial meats with obesity, diabetes, heart disease, cancers, neurological disorders, and chronic illness. In addition, these meats also contain antibiotics, hormones, pesticides, and herbicides.

Grass-fed and free-range meats, and wild-caught fish are safer. However, proteins from plant sources such as lentils, beans, green peas, quinoa, and amaranth are also great!

Six benefits of a healthy diet

- provides optimum nutrients
- reduces blood glucose
- decreases inflammation
- eliminates toxins
- heals the gut
- alkalizes the body[98]

Supplements

"Food is food, medicine is medicine, and both of them are really amazing."

~Dylan MacKay, Ph.D.

Most people in the United States take one or more dietary supplements either every day or occasionally. Dietary supplements include vitamins, minerals, protomorphogens, herbals and botanicals, amino acids, enzymes, and many other products. The most popular supplements include multivitamins especially vitamin B complex (make sure it's methylated if you have the MTHFR gene defect), vitamin D, and vitamin E, calcium, iron, probiotics, protein powders, omega-3 fish oils, glucosamine, turmeric, echinacea, and garlic.

The use of supplements is controversial. Many health professionals argue that supplements are unnecessary because we can get the essential nutrients we need from our diets alone. I have found that our food quality today just doesn't contain enough nutrients because of poor soil quality, GMO foods, pesticides, herbicides, and so on. Supplements help you to get adequate amounts of essential nutrients that may not be available in your diet, assuming your gut lining is in balance and you can absorb them properly. I do agree supplements can't replace the wide variety of foods in a healthy diet. Also, there is no consensus on the best supplements for overall health.[99] Your needs are as individualized as you are, and ever-changing.

Choosing the supplements that are right for you depend on your age, gender, diet, health status, genetics, and physical activity. For example, people who don't have enough exposure to sunlight may need more vitamin D. Vegetarians or vegans may need additional vitamin B12. Supplements should enhance and complement a balanced diet and a healthy lifestyle.[100]

The U.S. Food and Drug Administration (FDA) does not determine whether dietary supplements are effective before they are marketed. A supplement may not be safe just because it has a "natural" label. A supplement's safety depends on its chemical composition, how it is prepared, how it was stored, how it works in the body, and its dose. For example, herbs like comfrey and kava can harm the liver. So please, don't take any dietary supplement without consulting your health care provider.[101]

Clean water

"There's a very fundamental basic value system that I think America was built upon, and that's mutual respect, honor, integrity and concern for our environment and the right to clean water. And we have moved away from it."

~*Erin Brockovich*

Unfortunately, our tap water contains harmful substances like dangerous chemicals, compounds, and metals. A three-year study conducted by the Environmental Working Group throughout the country in 2009 found 316 chemicals in tap water. [102] Being from Flint, Michigan originally, I know firsthand about the Flint water crisis being contaminated with lead. Yes, that is an extreme toxicity but there are many chemicals found in our tap water that do more harm than good. For example, fluoride is a huge problem in the water supply of many cities. Fluoride negatively affects the thyroid causing it to shut down hormone production.

Contrary to popular belief, bottled water is not safe either. According to the National Resources Defense Council, 22 percent of the brands they tested contained contaminant levels above state health limits. Also, at least 25 percent of bottled water is just plain tap water.[103]

In addition, chemicals like Bisphenol A leach from the plastic bottles into the water causing hormone disruptions.

So, what is one to do? The safest option is to use a water filter at home such as a gravity filter that includes filtering out fluoride like Berkey or Propur, or reverse osmosis filters. They use a semi-permeable membrane that can trap any molecule larger than water. I promise[104] you will save so much money with a gravity filter versus buying bottled water, and you'll help save the environment as well!

How much water should you drink every day to prevent dehydration?

The answer is to drink about 50% of your body weight in ounces of water daily. If you weigh 140 pounds, drink about 70 ounces of water a day (about 2 liters). Additional ways to stay hydrated include eating more fruits and vegetables, using natural sea salt, and exercising regularly. Movement improves circulation and overall[105] electrolyte levels.[106]

Exercise

"If you only have time to exercise or meditate but not both, then make exercise your daily meditation."

~*Steve Pavlina*

Exercise is a natural way to relax, clear your mind, rejuvenate your body and helps to protect against the physical effects of daily stress. The benefits of regular exercise include:

- increases strength, flexibility and endurance
- strengthens bones and protects against osteoporosis
- reduces risk of heart disease[107]
- improves sleep[108]
- improves memory
- boosts energy and reduces fatigue[109]
- increases mood and self-confidence[110]
- improves work performance
- improves immunity[111]
- improves quality of life and lifespan[112]
- boosts happiness levels

Movement

"Lack of activity destroys the good condition of every human being, while movement and methodical physical exercise save it and preserve it."

~Plato

You may have heard that *sitting is the new smoking*. And most Americans have a sedentary job. Excessive sitting may shorten your lifespan—even if you go to the gym regularly![113] Paradoxically, increased movement helps to reduce the symptoms of fatigue and brain fog.

We need to move more and make movement a part of our lifestyle—whether it's walking, gardening, dancing, sports or taking the stairs instead of the elevator. One way to be more active is to exercise while watching TV. However, if you have been inactive for a while, consult your doctor before you start exercising.

Walking is a great place to start. If you are suffering with fatigue or pain, do not over due it. Start low and slow. Just walking 15-20 minutes a day is perfect. A rule of thumb is that if you are more fatigued after a workout, then it was too much. You have stressed your adrenal glands. You want to have a boost of energy after a workout. Ride those endorphins! If it's exhausting, it's too much stress on your body, for now.

Flow Yoga, Tai Chi, and **Pilates** are gentle forms of movement that are adaptable to any age and fitness level. Going to a regular class will help with accountability and building community, but you can also just pull up a YouTube vide and get started now.

Bodyweight exercises can be done in your office or home without any equipment. —all you need is your body. There are many varieties of these exercises and they can be adapted to any fitness level. Check out this article: *101 Bodyweight Exercises That You Can Do Anywhere* (http:// travelstrong.net/bodyweight-exercises/#).

Rebounders are mini-trampolines on which you can bounce or jog. Rebounding improves your physical fitness and also improves your lymphatic drainage, immune system, and bone strength. You can place it in your office or outdoors or in front of your TV. It's a great way for the family to exercise together.

Fitness trackers help to record and monitor your daily activity. Depending on your present level of fitness, you can set a daily goal of 1,000 steps or fewer and gradually increase it until you do 7,000 to 10,000 steps daily.

Fitness apps: There are some great fitness apps available today, and many are free.[114]

Charity Miles (https://charitymiles.org/) is a free app that donates money to the charity of your choice when you use it to log your running, walking or bicycling miles. For every mile you log, you help to earn money for your chosen charity. Corporate sponsors agree to donate a few cents for every mile you complete, and in exchange, they show you special offers in the app or otherwise expose you to their brands. The Charity Miles app lets anyone earn a little bit of money for a charity of their choice. It's available for both Android and iOS.

Spiritual practice – meditation

"Meditation: It's not what you think."

~*Dr. Jon Kabat-Zinn*

It is often said that meditation is to the mind what physical exercise is to the body. In fact, both exercise and meditation are beneficial for both mind and body.

Meditation means different things to different people. According to the Merriam-Webster Dictionary, meditation means to engage in a specific mental exercise or to focus one's thoughts on a specific object (such as concentration on one's breathing).[115]

Hundreds of clinical studies and trials have proved that meditation improves quality of life in various ways[116]:

- improves sleep quality
- improves response to chronic pain
- lowers inflammation
- boosts the immune system
- reduces headaches
- reduces overeating and risk of obesity
- helps people deal with chronic illnesses
- helps in mental disorders like eating disorders and bipolar disorder
- helps to deal with anxiety and depression

- lowers cortisol and stress levels
- helps with learning disabilities like ADHD and ADD
- improves decision-making and communication
- improves memory, focus, and mental clarity
- boosts effectiveness and efficiency at work
- increases positive feelings such as compassion, equanimity, happiness, and empathy[117]

Meditation has been used for centuries to heal both the body and mind in all religions and traditions. Like exercise, meditation can be done at home and even a few minutes of practice daily can be beneficial in several ways. Follow these tips to start your meditation practice:

- **Fix the time and place for your daily meditation:** Preferably first thing in the morning for a few minutes and a few minutes just before sleeping. Start small – set a timer of just 2-5 minutes and then gradually increase the time once you get used to this routine. Set a timer and sit until it goes off.
- **Use the right posture:** Initially, you can sit on a chair in an erect posture with your back straight but relaxed and eyes closed.
- **Give importance to the process, not the result:** During meditation, try to maintain a relaxed focus.

One effective way to do this is by experiencing the incoming and outgoing breath. When the mind wanders, as it will, sooner or later, smile and gently bring your attention back to your breath. And again. The goal is equanimity, not stillness of the mind (which is going to take a while). Gradually, you will learn to be aware of the reality of the present moment without any judgment or negative reaction.

Here's an exercise - For really active minds, I recommend a counting meditation. Take a deep breath in and hold it for the count of one, then let it out. Take another breath in and hold it for the count of two. Breathe in again and hold it for the count of three. Increase progressively and try to hold your breath up to a count of ten. If your mind starts to wander or you start thinking about the grocery list, start back over at one.

If you need support to start or maintain your meditation practice, check out the following sites:

- Ten Percent Happier:
  https://www.tenpercent.com/
- Calm: https://www.calm.com/
- Headspace: https://www.headspace.com/
- InsightTimer: https://insighttimer.com/

Annual labs with a functional practitioner

Has your primary care doctor told you, "All your blood tests look normal?" Or, "keep on doing what you're doing?" And have they said this in spite of your physical, mental or emotional complaints? If you keep on doing what you're doing, there is a chance that eventually even your basic labs will become abnormal!

Unfortunately, the current medical system does not focus on the prevention of disease. Primary care doctors often do not discuss lifestyle habits with their patients or prescribe extensive labs that can detect underlying dysfunction early enough to prevent serious illness. On the other hand, functional practitioners are more focused on detecting the early signs of dysfunction and preventing them before they become too serious.

The five types of blood tests you should do every year are:[118]

1. **Complete Blood Count and Complete Metabolic Panel**

   These two blood tests give information about your blood cell values, kidney function, liver function, and electrolyte and hydration status.

2. **Metabolic Markers: Fasting glucose, hemoglobin A1c, and lipid panel**

These metabolic markers help us to understand how you are processing macronutrients in the diet. Elevations in any of these levels can increase your risk for diabetes, heart disease, cancer, and Alzheimer's disease. Even if your Hba1c is in the normal range, every increase by 0.1 will increase the rate at which your brain shrinks in size per year.[119] Therefore, it is important to reach the optimal range, instead of staying in the normal range.

3. **Essential Nutrients: iron/ferritin, vitamin D, vitamin B12, magnesium**

Many people have deficiency of vitamin D, vitamin B12, iron, and magnesium, so they should be checked at least once a year. Again, it's important to consider their optimal range instead of the normal range. For example, the normal range of vitamin D may be from 30-100 nmol/L but the optimal range is 60-100 nmol/L.[120]

4. **Broad Thyroid Panel**

In most primary care clinics, only 1 or 2 thyroid markers are checked, usually TSH and/or total

T4. Six additional thyroid-related values need to be done: Total T3, Free T3, Reverse T3, T4, Free T4, Reverse T4, anti-TPO antibodies and anti-thyroglobulin antibodies. Also, the optimal range of values should be considered instead of the normal ranges of these labs. For example, the normal range for TSH is generally considered to be 0.2 – 4.5. However, some studies show that the body does not function properly when TSH rises above 2.5.[121]

5. **Inflammatory markers: homocysteine and CRP**

The blood level of C-reactive protein (CRP) increases when there's inflammation in the body. Even better, run a high-sensitivity C-reactive protein (hs-CRP). This test is more sensitive than a standard test. Even mild increases are associated with increased risk of cardiac events or depression.

Homocysteine is an amino acid that requires methylated-vitamin B12 and folate to be cleared. It's an important marker that can indicate vitamin B status, ability to methylate, ability to detox, risk of heart disease, risk of stroke, etc.

Be your own advocate

"I don't like to gamble, but if there's one thing I'm willing to bet on, it's myself."

~Beyoncé

Yes, I just quoted Beyoncé. Why? Because she's the Queen Bee of course!

I want to leave you with this. If there is one message you take from this book, let it be this. You are your best and only true advocate when it comes to your body, your mind, and your health. I have been there. I have sat in a doctor's office and was told I am fine. It's all in my head. Exercise more. Go home and get some rest. Or my favorite, stop worrying so much and you'll be fine.

Or worse, here is an antidepressant or pain medication, take this and be on your way. Remember, this was when I was only 15 years old. I was not was not lacking rest, I was not lacking exercise, I was not too worried, and I certainly was not depressed.

My body had broken down, and *I* needed to fix it. If your body is broken, and you know there is something wrong *DO NOT STOP* until you find the right team to help you fix it! You are the only one in your body. You are the only one who knows what it feels like when it is not functioning, don't let anyone convince you otherwise.

Doctors are just people, and they don't always have the answers. Some will dig deeper and some won't. We all take the oath to do no harm, and we try our best. But sometimes our best just isn't good enough. That's where *you* have to find the physician within you, and listen to your own voice. Find the team who will walk alongside you in your healing journey.

I pray you get the help you need and recover, like I did. Godspeed.

Next steps:

I believe that annual comprehensive lab tests, including genetic testing (genes only need to be run one time) can give us a complete picture of your health status. This enables us to advise you on the best and most effective way to regain optimal health and wellness. Lifestyle choices are an integral part of our holistic health approach as well as listening to your inner voice and your body.

Also, build your healing A-team!

TESTIMONIALS

Dr. Wards is a healer pure and simple. She listens to me and works with me. She doesn't talk down to me and makes use of my ideas if they make sense. She tells you what she can and can't do. She recommends other health practitioners if needed. She works on the most important issues and remembers the less important ones later on. She works in concert with my other health practitioners. She is always studying and learning new things to help her patients. She calls and follows up and takes the time to actually talk to me. She understands my healthcare is my responsibility and she helps me handle the responsibility in a very responsible way.

–DeeDee

Dr. Wards saved my life. She is the 25th health practitioner I've seen in my life for many, many health problems and no one has been able to help me heal food allergies, fatigue, sleep issues, etc. For at least the past 20 years I've eaten only organic food, no toxic anything in my life, and exercise 5 days per week, so I should be healthy as a horse.

–M

My first visit, she suspected a genetic defect and recommended lab work. It came back positive and the supplements have changed my life. No exaggeration, I had only felt good one day in my whole life before this and have now felt amazing for two weeks straight. Great energy level and positive outlook. She is a truly amazing health practitioner.

–A

I've started working with Dr. Wards two years into my health mess. I have a long list of issues: Lyme, methylation issues, adrenal issues, hormonal issues, POTS, etc. After only a couple of visits with her, I've seen a WORLD of improvement. She helped me sort out genetic methylation issues, even out my hormones, and calm my adrenals! I've been to several doctors and she's been incredible. Very thankful to be working with her! Staff is great also.

–Lindsey

I started seeing Dr. Wards 8 months ago. I was having anxiety and panic attacks. My primary care doctor prescribed me antidepressants which I chose not to take. After hormone and blood tests, Dr. Wards found that I have Hashimoto's and helped me change my diet and has guided me with a few supplements. My 2nd blood test after 6 months showed many improvements and I am feeling so much better than I was! No more Anxiety!! I'm so grateful for her help and would recommend her to anyone! Worth every penny!!!

–Stephanie

I can't say enough great things about Dr. T and her staff. I went to her for various reasons. A. I was having stomach issues. B. I wasn't sleeping well. And C. I couldn't lose weight. My main reason was the stomach issues. That's pretty much cleared up. I'm sleeping better than I have in years! And I lost 14 pounds so far! Only 8 more and I'll be at my goal weight. She's changed my way of eating, and I actually don't hate it or feel deprived. This is the most consistent I've ever eaten healthy in my life probably. She spends a lot of time with me, and never feel rushed. She's always on time. I am so thankful I went to her. It's changed my life for the better.

–Ashleigh

I was diagnosed two years with Celiac Disease. I immediately went gluten-free and began to feel much better. I continued to have other symptoms, including joint pain, shallow breathing, burning pain in my feet, general fatigue, irritability, insomnia, among others. I thought they were related to my Celiac Disease but just could not get better. I went to a number of traditional doctors (general practice, GI doc, rheumatologist, ENT, allergist, among others) and no one could really tell me what was wrong. It's so frustrating when you know your body and you know there is something wrong with you and medical professionals can do nothing to make you feel better and diagnose your problem. As a very active person (I work out once/twice per day), this was extremely concerning to me.

I took a chance and decided to go to Infinity Wellness Center. I saw Dr. Tenesha Wards, who was absolutely fabulous. She made me, finally, feel like I wasn't crazy. She spent more time talking to me and discussing my symptoms during the first visit than all of the western medicine doctors combined. I felt like she really listened and cared about putting a plan in place to get me feeling better.

After four months, I am finally at a point where I'm feeling "normal" again – like my old self. Through testing, acupuncture, genetic testing, and holistic supplements, I am now almost symptom free. I have worked in the medical field for 30 years so to finally get relief by seeking alternative care was a true stretch for me. If this is you, don't hesitate, do it. There is relief out there for you and it's with Dr. Wards. I highly recommend her and Infinity Wellness Center.

–Michael

I've been going to Infinity Wellness for many years and have had nothing by an amazing experience each time. After all this time, I would consider Dr. Wards a personal friend, and feel honored to do so! Nutrition, physiology, and mental perspective are all treated with equal care and attention.

–Meredith K

I highly recommend her to all my friends and anyone who is experiencing autoimmune disease, muscular or sports injuries or simple aches and pains of aging and living.

–Sallie

I came in with some kidney and bowel issues about 6 months ago. After a few cleanses and some great herbal supplements, I left my appointment today a different person. All of my symptoms have completely cleared up and I feel ten times better than when I came in. I did a GI cleanse, Candida cleanse, and kidney cleanse. They all worked wonders and it doesn't hurt that I also dropped a whole pant size :)

–E

I have been going to Dr. Wards for about 5 months now and I have noticed a drastic improvement in my specific areas of concern as well as my overall health!

I had been struggling with stomach problems for about 6 years now and traditional medicine had not delivered the results I had hoped so I tried Infinity Wellness and no longer have many of the digestive issues I care in with!

Even my other health challenges like migraine or painful cycle (which I had chalked up to being untreatable) were carefully examined and cared for. I appreciate how thoughtful Dr. Wards is and open to listen to any reaction or concern no matter how seemingly small.

Moral of the story, the whole team is great and I have referred one of my friends with an autoimmune disease and she has had equal success! Can't recommend her enough!

–Amy W.

HEALTH IS THE NEW WEALTH

"The great pharaohs of Egypt have been found in their tombs surrounded by glittering gold, sparkling jewels and the finest resources the world had to offer. Yet, each of them would have rather enjoyed an extra dozen healthy years living in the Egyptian sunshine. There is no amount of wealth that will make up for an early passing or lifetime of disease."

~Dr. George Birnbach

Congratulations on finishing the book! Whether you read every chapter or read the topics that were of interest to you, you are taking action. You rock!

Nine out of ten people who purchase books don't finish them. So, you are in the tiny minority of people who have decided to take charge of your health and seek information and help. That is the first right step.

Some of the important health principles in this book are:

- repair of the gut, detoxification pathways, endocrine system and nervous system
- protection and treatment of toxicity, infections, molds, allergies, and stress
- prevention and treatment of chronic inflammation
- strengthening of the immune system and correction of genetic variations
- importance of healthy food, clean water, appropriate supplements, regular exercise, movement, and meditation

The most important takeaway is that you have to take responsibility for your own health and wellness. As I explained at the start of this book, our conventional medical system is not fully equipped to deal with conditions like Lyme Disease, leaky gut syndrome, food allergies, other stealth infections, and adrenal fatigue.

Though there's a lot of information in this book, it's not possible to include all the information you need. Also, health books like this one have limitations because each person is different with individual health issues determined by their genes, environment, age, gender, emotions, and past illnesses.

I hope this book was helpful to you. If you have any questions or comments, please email me at dr.tenesha@austinholisticdr.com. I'd love to hear about your health stories.

All the best for your onward journey to a vibrant and healthy life. JUST KEEP GOING!

With lots of gratitude,

Dr. Tenesha

ABOUT THE AUTHOR

Dr. Tenesha Wards is a graduate of Texas Chiropractic College and founder of The Energy Recovery System online health coaching program and Infinity Wellness Center, located in Austin, Texas. She has completed certifications in Genetic Sciences, Acupuncture, Applied Kinesiology, Activator Technique, Webster Technique and Applied Clinical Nutrition.

Dr. Wards' personal struggle with Lyme disease, EBV, and autoimmunity fuel her passion for a holistic approach to wellness. Overcoming her debilitating health experiences gave her the empathy to relate to her patients. She believes in the importance of treating the whole person and not just the symptoms.

Dr. Wards practices holistically, specializing in determining the underlying causes of conditions such as exhaustion, burnout, chronic pain, fibromyalgia, and headaches.

Dr. Wards' work is based on a fundamental principle that promoting health and wellness has no boundary. From earthquake relief work in Haiti to cancer survivors in Guadalajara, Dr. Wards is committed to not just practicing locally, but globally. In addition to promoting health and wellness of the body, Dr. Wards also supports her community through leadership roles with the Texas Women in Business, Westlake Chamber of Commerce and philanthropic service with the Center for Child Protection and Mobile Loaves and Fishes.

Dr. Wards also keeps up on the latest postgraduate training classes to ensure her patients receive the most advanced care. Dr. Wards has traveled all over the nation learning from the top doctors in the country and mastering the most advanced methods of drug-free healthcare. She has studied under Dr. Evan Mladdenoff, team physician for the Kansas City Chiefs, Drs. George and Jeannette Birnbach, pioneers in clinical nutrition and advanced clinical therapy, Dr. John Bandy, Lance Armstrong's kinesiologist, Dr. Stuart White, one of the leading clinical nutritionists, and Dr. Kendal Stewart, neurotologist and neuroimmune specialist focusing on genetic defects.

Most recently, she has added Autonomic Response testing to her toolbox, studying under Dr. Klinghardt, who is featured in the documentary on Lyme disease *"Under Our Skin"*.

Considered an expert in functional blood lab ranges, Dr. Wards has taught an ongoing study group in her office, sponsored by Apex Energetics teaching functional nutrition to other doctors.

Many people come to Dr. Wards after experiencing a lack of results with traditional practitioners and cookie-cutter programs. Her success is based on the ability to discover the root cause of a patient's symptoms, and then to design a custom program based on their body's chemistry, resulting in restored energy and a renewed enthusiasm for life!

If you are not in Texas, you can work with Dr. Wards in her online program.

The Energy Recovery System

Website: www.Energy-Recovery-System.com

Instagram: https://www.instagram.com/energy_recovery_system/

Facebook: https://www.facebook.com/energyrecoverysystem/

Dr. Tenesha Wards, D.C., A.C.N.

Email: dr.tenesha@austinholisticdr.com

Get Connected:

Here are her social media links:

Instagram: https://www.instagram.com/drtenesha/

LinkedIn: https://www.linkedin.com/in/drtenesha/

YouTube: https://www.youtube.com/user/drteneshaweine

Facebook: https://www.facebook.com/Dr.TeneshaWeine

Infinity Wellness Center

1201 West Slaughter Lane Austin, Texas 78748

Website: https://www.austinholisticdr.com

Phone: (512) 328-0505

Fax: (512) 291-7702

Email: info@austinholisticdr.com

Facebook: https://www.facebook.com/InfinityWellnessATX/

Instagram: https://www.instagram.com/infinitywellnessatx/

To book an appointment, go to https://nutralysiswellness.com/landing/infinitywellness

ENDNOTES

1. http://www.ncbi.nlm.nih.gov/pmc/articles/PMC3426293/
2. https://www.ncbi.nlm.nih.gov/pubmed/29701810
3. http://www.ncbi.nlm.nih.gov/pmc/articles/PMC3897394/
4. http://www.hopkinsmedicine.org/health/healthy_aging/healthy_
    body/the-brain-gut-connection
5. https://www.ncbi.nlm.nih.gov/pmc/articles/PMC4316216/
6. https://www.ncbi.nlm.nih.gov/pmc/articles/PMC2551660/
7. https://www.health.harvard.edu/blog/leaky-gut-what-is-it-and-
    what-does-it-mean-for-you-2017092212451
8. https://www.ncbi.nlm.nih.gov/pubmed/7714684
9. http://www.ncbi.nlm.nih.gov/pmc/articles/PMC3458511/
10. https://www.holistichelp.net/organic-acids-test.html
11. https://draxe.com/leaky-gut-diet-treatment/
12. https://www.ncbi.nlm.nih.gov/pubmed/25972430
13. https://www.ncbi.nlm.nih.gov/pmc/articles/PMC4518423/
14. http://www.ncbi.nlm.nih.gov/pubmed/2345464
15. https://www.bbc.com/news/world-us-canada-43050394
16. https://www.niddk.nih.gov/health-information/diabetes/
    preventing-diabetes-problems/low-blood-glucose-
    hypoglycemiadiabetes or prediabetes

17. https://www.merckmanuals.com/en-pr/home/digestive-disorders/biology-of-the-digestive-system/pancreas
18. https://www.diabetes.co.uk/body/endocrine-system.html
19. https://www.merckmanuals.com/home/hormonal-and-metabolic-disorders/diabetes-mellitus-dm-and-disorders-of-blood-sugar-metabolism/diabetes-mellitus-dm
20. National Diabetes Statistics Report, 2017. Centers for Disease Control and Prevention website. https://www.cdc.gov/diabetes/data/statistics/statistics-report.html
21. https://dtc.ucsf.edu/types-of-diabetes/type2/understanding-type-2-diabetes/how-the-body-processes-sugar/blood-sugar-stress/
22. https://www.merckmanuals.com/home/hormonal-and-metabolic-disorders/diabetes-mellitus-dm-and-disorders-of-blood-sugar-metabolism/diabetes-mellitus-dm
23. https://www.merckmanuals.com/home/hormonal-and-metabolic-disorders/diabetes-mellitus-dm-and-disorders-of-blood-sugar-metabolism/hypoglycemia
24. https://www.diabetes.co.uk/what-is-hba1c.html
25. https://www.merckmanuals.com/home/hormonal-and-metabolic-disorders/diabetes-mellitus-dm-and-disorders-of-blood-sugar-metabolism/diabetes-mellitus-dm#v773034
26. https://www.ncbi.nlm.nih.gov/pmc/articles/PMC3977406/
27. https://www.merckmanuals.com/home/hormonal-and-metabolic-disorders/diabetes-mellitus-dm-and-disorders-of-blood-sugar-metabolism/diabetes-mellitus-dm
28. https://www.thelancet.com/journals/lancet/article/PIIS0140-6736(17)33102-1/fulltext
29. https://www.ncbi.nlm.nih.gov/pubmed/23678828
30. https://www.ncbi.nlm.nih.gov/pubmed/24019277
31. https://www.ncbi.nlm.nih.gov/pmc/articles/PMC4027280/
32. https://www.ncbi.nlm.nih.gov/pubmed/17109600
33. https://www.ncbi.nlm.nih.gov/pmc/articles/PMC3430014/
34. https://www.ncbi.nlm.nih.gov/pmc/articles/PMC4583053/

35. https://www.ncbi.nlm.nih.gov/pubmed/16401645
36. https://www.ncbi.nlm.nih.gov/pmc/articles/PMC2992225/
37. http://academic.brooklyn.cuny.edu/biology/bio4fv/page/ph_def.htm
38. https://www.merckmanuals.com/home/hormonal-and-metabolic-disorders/acid-base-balance/overview-of-acid-base-balance
39. https://www.ncbi.nlm.nih.gov/pubmed/20003625
40. https://www.ncbi.nlm.nih.gov/pmc/articles/PMC2803035/
41. https://www.ncbi.nlm.nih.gov/pubmed/25037581
42. Baroody T.A. (2015) *Alkalize or Die.* (11th ed.) Waynesville, NC: Holographic Health Press
43. https://www.ncbi.nlm.nih.gov/pmc/articles/PMC3195546/
44. https://upload.wikimedia.org/wikipedia/commons/c/c6/Illu_endocrine_system.jpg
45. https://www.merckmanuals.com/home/hormonal-and-metabolic-disorders/biology-of-the-endocrine-system/endocrine-glands
46. https://www.merckmanuals.com/home/hormonal-and-metabolic-disorders/biology-of-the-endocrine-system/endocrine-function
47. https://www.merckmanuals.com/home/hormonal-and-metabolic-disorders/biology-of-the-endocrine-system/endocrine-function
48. https://www.merckmanuals.com/home/hormonal-and-metabolic-disorders/biology-of-the-endocrine-system/endocrine-disorders
49. https://www.merckmanuals.com/home/hormonal-and-metabolic-disorders/biology-of-the-endocrine-system/effects-of-aging-on-the-endocrine-system
50. https://draxe.com/10-ways-balance-hormones-naturally/
51. https://www.tgh.org/services/diabetes-endocrinology/endocrine-disorders-testing-and-diagnosis
52. https://medlineplus.gov/lab-tests/cortisol-test/
53. https://www.diagnostechs.com/our-tests/adrenal-stress-index-asi/
54. https://www.zrtlab.com/sample-types/saliva/
55. https://draxe.com/hyperthyroidism-vs-hypothyroidism/
56. https://labtestsonline.org/conditions/pituitary-disorders
57. http://www.ncbi.nlm.nih.gov/pmc/articles/PMC1524969/

58. http://www.ncbi.nlm.nih.gov/pmc/articles/PMC1592668/

59. https://www.merckmanuals.com/professional/endocrine-and-metabolic-disorders/principles-of-endocrinology/overview-of-endocrine-disorders

60. http://www.ncbi.nlm.nih.gov/pmc/articles/PMC3573577/

61. https://draxe.com/10-ways-balance-hormones-naturally/

62. http://www.downeshealth.com/blogs/Protomorphogens.php

63. https://www.niehs.nih.gov/health/topics/agents/endocrine/index.cfm

64. http://www.atsdr.cdc.gov/emes/public/docs/Chemicals,%20Cancer,%20and%20You%20FS.pdf

65. https://www.ncbi.nlm.nih.gov/pubmed/20806995

66. http://www.cdc.gov/biomonitoring/pdf/FourthReport_UpdatedTables_Feb2015.pdf

67. https://www.merriam-webster.com/dictionary/toxin

68. https://www.merriam-webster.com/dictionary/free%20radical

69. https://www.ncbi.nlm.nih.gov/pubmed/8221017

70. Phillips, T. (2008). The role of methylation in gene expression. Nature Education, 1(1), 116

71. http://www.dietvsdisease.org/mthfr-mutation-symptoms-and-diet/

72. http://mthfr.net/mthfr-mutations-and-the-conditions-they-cause/2011/09/07/

73. https://medlineplus.gov/liverfunctiontests.html

74. https://medlineplus.gov/lab-tests/ast-test/

75. https://medlineplus.gov/lab-tests/alt-blood-test/

76. https://labtestsonline.org/tests/gamma-glutamyl-transferase-ggt

77. https://draxe.com/fighting-free-radical-damage/

78. https://draxe.com/detox-diet/

79. https://rawlsmd.com/health-articles/what-is-a-stealth-microbe

80. Dr. Evan H. Hirsch. Fix Your Fatigue. 2017

81. https://bengreenfieldfitness.com/article/digestion-articles/blame-bugs-stealth-pathogens-making-fat-tired-brain-dead/

82. https://www.cdc.gov/drugresistance/index.html

83. https://www.ncbi.nlm.nih.gov/pubmed/15886693

84. Cook GC, Zumla AI (2008). *Manson's Tropical Diseases: Expert Consult*. Edinburgh, Scotland: Saunders Ltd. p. 347. ISBN 978-1-4160-4470-3

85. https://www.cdc.gov/parasites/about.html

86. http://www.ncbi.nlm.nih.gov/pubmedhealth/PMHT0025348/

87. https://draxe.com/lyme-disease-symptoms/

88. http://www.cdc.gov/lyme/

89. http://cid.oxfordjournals.org/content/31/4/1107.long

90. http://www.tickencounter.org/prevention/protect_yourself

91. https://www.merckmanuals.com/professional/infectious-diseases/herpesviruses/overview-of-herpesvirus-infections

92. https://www.cdc.gov/epstein-barr/about-ebv.html

93. https://www.cdc.gov/epstein-barr/laboratory-testing.html

94. https://www.cdc.gov/fungal/diseases/candidiasis/index.html

95. https://draxe.com/candida-symptoms/

96. https://draxe.com/candida-symptoms/

97. https://onlinelibrary.wiley.com/doi/full/10.1111/j.1365-3083.2010.02458.x

98. https://draxe.com/healing-diet/

99. https://ods.od.nih.gov/HealthInformation/DS_WhatYouNeedToKnow.aspx

100. https://draxe.com/best-supplements/

101. https://ods.od.nih.gov/HealthInformation/DS_WhatYouNeedToKnow.aspx

102. http://www.ewg.org/tap-water/

103. https://www.nrdc.org/stories/truth-about-tap

104. https://draxe.com/tap-water-toxicity/

105. https://draxe.com/how-to-stay-hydrated/

106. http://www.ncbi.nlm.nih.gov/pubmed/11539751

107. http://www.bmj.com/content/347/bmj.f5577

108. http://www.aasmnet.org/jcsm/ViewAbstract.aspx?pid=29078

109. http://well.blogs.nytimes.com/2008/02/29/the-cure-for-exhaustion-more-exercise/

110. http://news.ufl.edu/archive/2009/10/uf-study-exercise-improves-body-image-for-fit-and-unfit-alike.html

111. http://www.nlm.nih.gov/medlineplus/ency/article/007165.htm

112. http://journals.plos.org/plosmedicine/article?id=10.1371/journal.pmed.1001335

113. U.S. Department of Health and Human Services. Physical Activity and Health: A Report of the Surgeon General. Atlanta: Centers for Disease Control and Prevention; 1996

114. Dr. Evan H. Hirsch. Fix Your Fatigue. 2017

115. https://www.merriam-webster.com/dictionary/meditate

116. https://www.ncbi.nlm.nih.gov/pubmed/24395196

117. https://draxe.com/guided-meditation/

118. https://www.parsleyhealth.com/blog/5-essential-blood-tests-need-every-year/

119. http://n.neurology.org/content/64/10/1704.long

120. https://www.ncbi.nlm.nih.gov/pmc/articles/PMC4015454/

121. https://www.ncbi.nlm.nih.gov/pubmed/20534758

Made in the USA
Coppell, TX
29 September 2021

63194699R00085